I0116808

a little handbook about

addiction

AND THE FUTURE OF RECOVERY
THAT COULD INCLUDE CANNABIS

kayla fioravanti &
keegan fioravanti

EPILOGUE BY CARLTON BONE

Selah
Press
PUBLISHING

A Little Handbook About Addiction and the Future of Recovery That Could Include Cannabis

By Kayla Fioravanti and Keegan Fioravanti
Editor: Venessa Knizley
Cover Design: Haleigh Fioravanti
Copyright © 2019 Kayla Fioravanti and Keegan Fioravanti

ISBN: 978-1-7343016-0-1

Printed in the United States of America, Published by Selah Press
For information on getting permission for reprints and excerpts, contact:
kayla@kaylafioravanti.com

Printed in the United States of America, Published by Selah Press

Notice of Rights: All rights reserved. No part of this book may be reproduced or transmitted in any form by any means, electronic, mechanical, photocopy, recording or other without the prior written permission of the publisher.

For information on getting permission for reprints and excerpts, contact: kayla@ologyessentials.com

Notice of Liability: The author has made every effort possible to check and ensure the accuracy of the information and recipes presented in this book. However, the information herein is sold without warranty, either expressed or implied. The author, publisher nor any dealer or distributor of this book will be held liable for any damages caused either directly or indirectly by the instructions, recipes or information contained in this book.

Disclaimer: Information in this book is NOT intended as medical advice, nor for use as diagnosis or treatment of a health problem, nor as a substitute for consulting a licensed medical professional. The contents and information in this book are for informational use only and are not intended to be a substitute for professional medical advice, diagnosis or treatment. Always seek the advice of your physician or other qualified health provider for medical conditions. Never disregard professional medical advice or delay in seeking it because of something you read in this book or any resource.

Dedication

From Kayla

To my dad for showing me the way to sobriety by battling and destroying the beast before my very young eyes. Your health journey has been an inspiration and road map—you are my hero.

From Keegan

To my wife Haleigh for showing me pure happiness in living your life. You have given me the strength to face my demons and come out the other end a stronger man. To my everything!

Contents

Introduction

"Your assumptions are your windows on the world. Scrub them off every once in a while, or the light won't come in." Isaac Asimov

Keegan and I wrote this little book to start the conversation about addiction and substance abuse and how hemp CBD may play a role in the future of treatment options. It is not meant to be the be all and end all on the subject. The use of hemp CBD for addiction is an emerging field.

Honestly, I was skeptical about the benefits of hemp CBD in general at first. And, well, if I'm totally honest, I was inclined to believe that hemp CBD was just another fad in the natural industry. But my son, Keegan, kept telling me to try it, and I figured it would be easier to try it because he was never going to stop asking me to. I wouldn't say I'm a pessimist when it comes to new natural products, but I am someone who wants to see the science—more of a questioner would be the best way to describe me. Since I've been in the natural industry since 1998, I just assumed it was another product that had some value but could not possibly be the natural wonder that people were making it out to be.

The cannabis plant has given me the ability to live a life without prescriptions and constant physical pain. I was determined to show my mother this beautiful plant to help her live the same life. ~Keegan

My son is persistent, so I started digging. I saw that a chemist who I've known and trusted for nearly twenty years was doing some testing for a lab in the hemp CBD industry. I figured if I was going to start anywhere, I'd start looking in the direction that someone I trusted was working. So I ordered some samples of full spectrum hemp CBD oil for internal use.

I didn't have time to do any research before my samples arrived, so I just blindly followed the directions on the bottle, which is an anomaly for me. I thought that maybe the hemp CBD might help with the chronic joint pain that had plagued me for my whole life. I had only recently discovered that the pain was a symptom of Ehler's Danlos Syndrome, a genetic connective tissue disorder.

After a day, I discovered that I didn't need to take the anti-inflammatories that had become part of my daily routine. That seemed promising. The next day I felt even better and on the third day, the symptoms that were about to force me to have a hysterectomy had completely resolved. *Wait! What?* I had tried every option medicine had to offer to resolve those symptoms, including aromatherapy, herbs, diet, exercise, traditional medicine and a year of prayers, with absolutely no relief. I had not even for a moment thought that three days of taking hemp CBD would help me avoid the dreaded hysterectomy I had finally accepted as inevitable.

I called Keegan and told him that I was a hemp CBD believer, and I was ready to jump into the industry headfirst with my son and daughter-in-law—hence, Ology Essentials was born. I dove deep into the research to understand why hemp CBD actually *was* nature's amazing wonder drug.

One of the nagging questions that also had made me drag my feet on the whole idea of hemp CBD was my own misconception that hemp was so closely related to marijuana that there could be safety or addiction concerns for me. I've been sober since February 1992. I did not want to expose myself to anything that could jeopardize my sobriety or anyone else's for that matter. I am thrilled to tell you that hemp CBD is completely safe, and I will address that concern in greater detail in Chapter 2. I am all too aware of my own addictive tendencies and want to be sensitive to others like me.

The key to understanding why hemp CBD is not an addictive is the fact that it does not release excessive levels of dopamine into the brain. Instead of getting you high, hemp CBD works to create a balanced level of neurotransmitter into the brain. I can personally attest to hemp CBD being non-addictive, but honestly, you deserve more. In December 2017 the World Health Organization's Expert Committee on Drug Dependence came out with a statement declaring that cannabidiol (CBD) is not an addictive chemical and poses no threat to public health. The World Health Organization (WHO) also suggested that there is no scientific basis for prohibiting cannabidiol.

The report declared that not only is CBD not addictive, it also shows promising potential for addicts: "Another possible therapeutic application which has been investigated is the use of CBD to treat drug addiction. A recent systematic review concluded that there were a limited number of preclinical studies which suggest that CBD may have therapeutic properties on opioid, cocaine, and psychostimulant addiction, and some preliminary data suggest that it may be beneficial in cannabis and tobacco addiction in humans"[1]

Some worry that there hasn't been enough research into the safety of hemp CBD. However, I found countless studies *and* even studies of studies. An example of this thorough research was done by Mateus Machado Bergamashci who completed a comprehensive survey of the safety and side effects of CBD using reports retrieved from *Web of Science, Scielo and Medline*. His research, "Safety and Side Effects of Cannabidiol, a Cannabis sativa Constituent," was published in *Current Drug Safety*. Bergamashci found that CBD is safe for humans and animals.[2]

In 2011, Iffland Kerstin and Grotenhermen Franjo from the German research center nova-Institut set out to expand on Bergamaschci's findings with a new comprehensive study, "An Update on Safety and Side Effects of Cannabidiol: A Review of Clinical Data and Relevant Animal Studies." Kerstin and Franjo's studies found that CBD had no adverse effect on blood pressure, heart rate, body temperature, glucose levels, pH, pressure exerted by carbon dioxide or oxygen, hematocrits, gastrointestinal transit, emesis, rectal temperature, potassium and sodium levels, and no reparatory depression or cardiovascular complications. The study also found that even chronic use of CBD in humans caused no neurological, psychiatric or clinical adverse effects. In even more positive news, the new study found CBD is potentially beneficial in the treatment of heroin addiction, reducing seizures, managing psychosis, inhibiting cancer and reducing anxiety. They also found that cannabinoid has immunomodulatory and neuroprotective properties.[3] This is of no surprise, since the American government obtained a patent in 1998 for cannabinoids as antioxidants and neuroprotectants.[4]

Iffland and Grotenhermen also found that hemp CBD has a better side effect profile for the treatment of epilepsy and psychotic disorders, which they believed could improve the compliance and adherence to treatment.[5] Anyone who has ever suffered through the side effects of any over-the-counter or prescription drug knows exactly how important this finding is for hemp CBD to be used as an alternative therapy for multiple diseases and disorders.

Iffland and Grotenhermen went on to state that, "At lower doses, it [CBD] has physiological effects that promote and

4

maintain health, including antioxidative, anti-inflammatory, and neuroprotection effects. For instance, CBD is more effective than vitamin C and E as a neuroprotective antioxidant and can ameliorate skin conditions such as acne."[6]

Once upon a time, marijuana was viewed as a gateway drug; however, many now believe it to be an exit drug. This book is about hemp CBD, but you will see some information on how legalized marijuana has impacted the opioid crisis in certain states. We are not advising or endorsing the use of either hemp or marijuana in place of medical treatment for substance abuse disorder, mental health, or any other medical condition. To reiterate our disclaimer: Information in this book is NOT intended as medical advice, nor for use as diagnosis or treatment of a health problem, nor as a substitute for consulting a licensed medical professional. The contents and information in this book are for informational use only and are not intended to be a substitute for professional medical advice, diagnosis or treatment. Always seek the advice of your physician or other qualified health provider for medical conditions. Never disregard professional medical advice or delay in seeking it because of something you read in this book or any resource.

Chapter 1
Our Personal Battles

"You cannot find peace by avoiding life." Virginia Woolf

Kayla's Story

I am probably the most unlikely candidate to jump on the hemp CBD oil bandwagon. And yet, here I am. My family's multi-generational struggle impacted me with direct hits as the child of an alcoholic, as an alcoholic myself and as the mother of an addict. The word *cannabis* was deeply woven in my mind with marijuana—and for me that was something I didn't want to get involved in. My son's insistence that I look into hemp CBD sent me digging for information, which I share in detail in Chapter 2.

My own drinking began in sixth grade—at twelve years old. I lived overseas on a military base called McGraw Kaserne in the American housing area known as Perlacher Forst in Munich, Germany. Beer was abundantly available on and off base. Cheap American beer could be purchased in unattended vending machines that I could ride my bike or walk to all over Perlacher Forst and McGraw Kaserne. The Germans also would sell beer to us off base, which was just a hop-skip-and-a-jump from just about anywhere my friends and I might have been on base. Additionally, everyone's parents had large stashes of good German beer that we could pilfer without anyone ever noticing.

When we drank the cheap American beer from the vending machines, we used to keep wintergreen mints in our mouth to combat the foul, watered-down taste—drunkenness was the goal. Everyone enjoyed the good German beer. At first, we hid away in Perlacher Forest to drink our treasures, but over time, we became bold and drank at the local German restaurants and pubs. In sixth and seventh grade, we drank to be cool and part of the culture around us. In seventh grade, my gymnastic teacher introduced us to a kind of schnapps known as Apfelkorn. It soon became a favorite treat.

Studies have shown that people who start drinking before age fifteen are four times more likely to develop alcohol dependence at some time in their lives compared with those who have their first drink at age twenty or older.[1] Well, starting to drink at twelve, and coming from a long line of alcoholics, was the perfect combination for me to develop an early and serious addiction.

Despite my drinking, I excelled in sports and academics. I moved to America in eight grade and lead the party scene solidly through two more moves. I drowned multiple hurts in booze and dealt with the stress of moving in eighth and eleventh grade by avoiding it all through drunkenness. I didn't adjust well to only having American beer available, so I moved onto Vodka, EverClear and Tequila as my staples.

In college, I was right at home in the party scene. I never just hung out with one group of friends; I had many different groups of friends to cover my problem. Not everyone was up to drinking every night of the week, but I was so diversified with my friendships that there was always at least one friend to drink with, if not an entire party to participate in.

Ironically, I majored in psychology with an emphasis on addiction. I worked internships to help other hurting people get sober, all while being a hurting person who was avoiding reality and sobriety. During my senior year of college, I worked as a drug and alcohol counselor at a large public high school. The kids who I was leading in an addiction group challenged me to be sober with them. I never confessed to having a problem, but they figured if they couldn't drink, then I should take the challenge with them. I took them up on it. I spent the last few months of college sober. I was twenty-two, and it was the first time I'd been sober for any period of time since I was twelve years old.

I was living like a manic depressive—happy one moment until the next wave hit when I became dark and remorseful. I had been self-medicating for 10 years—sobriety was hard. At graduation, someone handed me a glass of champagne. I rationalized that it was okay to take one drink because I had just graduated with honors and even made the Dean's list after all. I remember that it was a rainy wet day in Portland, Oregon, when I graduated. I remember my brother popping a champagne bottle as we stood under a tree posing for pictures. I wondered, *What harm can a glass of champagne do?*

I partook in the celebration, toasting with champagne. And with that, my first bout of sobriety ended. I spiraled right back into being a full-blown alcoholic. I was in a super unhealthy place in life—days were brittle and nights were stone cold. I was running with booze as my crutch.

Suddenly, I was now a grown up and completely on my own for the first time. My life had been stained with a badge of victimhood, and I still wore it daily. I had taken to heart the messages of those who filled my mind with confusing and disorienting messages. I partied even harder to cope.

The party train abruptly ended when I was twenty-four years old. One morning, with no memory of the night before, I awoke feeling life inside of me. The feeling of life was foreign and altogether consuming, as I had been so dead and so numb for so very long. I knew with certainty that I was pregnant. Just as suddenly, I also knew I had to protect this new life with all of my being.

I was only hours pregnant when I chose to stop drinking for the good of my child. I had studied fetal alcohol syndrome in college. I couldn't bear to injure this baby. I was willing and ready to sacrifice everything to protect my child. My future plans to obtain my Ph.D. were quickly abandoned. They now become meaningless in the face of this new life.

I went to the store a week later to buy a pregnancy test and bottle of wine. I decided one or the other would be my future. The test came up positive, so I gave the bottle of wine to my neighbors. I went into town to get an official test run. I remember clearly walking the streets of Portland after getting the news, with no idea how I was going stand up to the burden of the challenge ahead of me. I quickly learned that I would be parenting alone.

I was violently ill from both the pregnancy and alcohol withdraws. It was hard to think, but I knew that having this baby would somehow save my life. I didn't know how, but I knew this child was a life preserver. I was willing and able to let go of the future I had planned to grasp hold of the hope of a new future. With my love for my child solidified in my heart, everything changed. I discovered a love bigger than I ever imagined possible as I faced pregnancy alone.

My parents were devastated by the news of my pregnancy. The hardest phone call I ever had to make was the international call to Germany to tell them that I was pregnant. I sat on my futon listening to the unique sound of an international ring and gathered up my courage.

My mom answered, "Well hello, Kayla," in her familiar sing song voice.

I had to break her joy of hearing from me with difficult news.

My mom informed me, "You can't come home."

I replied, "I know."

I knew because my parents had been preparing me my whole life to live independently, to live with the consequences of my choices and to stand on my own two feet. There was no resentment between us as she let me know that door was closed.

During my pregnancy, I cried more tears than I knew my body could produce. I was terrified. I was ill-equipped for motherhood, and I knew it. In addition, I was facing this difficult challenge sober. After giving birth when they set my son on my stomach, I wept. And for the first time in nine months, they were tears of joy. I was swept with an overwhelming love beyond anything I could have ever imagined. I had thought I knew what love was, but I was wrong. I only knew the outside edges of love until I became a mother. My love for my son, Keegan, was bigger than anything I could have ever dreamed.

I felt like I was born the day my son was born. A whole new life opened up to me with new emotions. Motherhood expanded my heart. It opened me up to feel everything. All the parts of me that I had closed swung open in the first moments of motherhood. I knew my son was a life preserver thrown to me by someone bigger than I could imagine.

I got sober to protect my son while he grew inside of me— I stayed sober to protect my son from the emotional damage I knew I would inflict on him if I remained an active alcoholic. Today, I stay sober for me. I don't want to miss anything. I have three adult children, and with each, I have learned deeper levels of love as I walk beside them.

Keegan's Story

It is always so wild for me to hear my mother's story of addiction. As a child, I would have never guessed it because she was so strait-laced and such a go-getter. Addiction was not brought up much in our family as I grew up, but it was known in the family that we had a long line of addiction problems. I was, and am, a very strong minded individual, and back then, I didn't think it would ever affect me. I was incredibly naive.

Growing up with my single mom, who had so much love and attention for me, made me want to do the same for her. I always wanted to make sure I was working as hard as her to keep us afloat, even though I didn't really know what that meant. If I could make her day easier by cleaning or doing any chores I could, I would help; we were a team. When I was six, my mother got married.

My path to substances abuse started with kind of a hilarious mess up on my parents account. I was sent to an entrepreneur leadership high school. It was a startup school, and I was in the first ever class. It turned out that all of the kids had been kicked out of private and public schools were able to get into this school. To put it blatantly, I was thrown into the belly of the beast, and because I had been pushed forward in school, I was only 11 going into my freshman year of high school.

I made friends very quickly and was introduced to opiates, xanax, hallucinogens, cocaine and alcohol within my first week of attending. My parents saw this very quickly. They saw the kids I went to school with and saw my change in attitude. So, they quickly transferred me to a private school in Portland, but I'd been given a taste of numbness. I moved to another school but kept my connections to the kids at the previous school. I would skip classes or leave early to meet them in the park behind my new school to get my fix in. I wasn't much of a partier. Once in a while, I would go out with a group of friends and indulge, but I was much less social with my addictions. Everyone knew something was going on, but no one knew the extent of what I was doing.

I had been working for my parent's business for years at their factory, so I always had money. By fourteen, I was popping every pill I could get my hands on, and I started to sell whatever I could to get more. I was cheating in school, stealing all of the time—in fact, I was stealing teacher textbooks, copying them and selling the copies. I was always scheming and lying to get my next fix. It all came to a head when I finally snapped and got myself expelled from my high school. After that, everything went downhill. I was caught and arrested a couple weeks later for shoplifting alcohol and snacks. I was coked out of my mind with no cares about anything, but I will never forget my mother's face when she picked me up from the station.

From there, my parents had to make a hard choice—either send me away to a program or watch me kill myself. Sadly, a lot of these programs that sell you on success rates don't actually do what they tell you they are going to do. They are mostly a scam. I say this from being in one for 10 months and talking with hundreds of kids and adults who have participated in similar programs. I came out of that program knowing how to manipulate the system better than I had ever before. I now had contacts all around America to get involved in the worst things possible.

Two months after getting out of rehab, I was back on the train of addiction. I had never really stopped; I was just waiting for everyone to stop watching me. From there, I went even farther off the deep end. I was seventeen and immersed in the drug world more than ever. I left Portland as soon as I could and moved to Hawaii with a girl I had met from rehab in Utah. This is where I lost it all.

It was almost two years of constant substance abuse. I was maybe only sober for 10 minutes a day, and that was the time I spent getting up in the morning. I had an endless supply and no intentions of quitting. I had multiple near-death experiences, overdoses and guns being pulled on me at drug deals.

None of these stopped me from keeping the train rolling until the night I pulled the dumbest move of all. I jumped onto a moving car and held on until it reached over 40 miles per hour before I was forced off the vehicle headfirst into the concrete. It was 3 a.m. in the morning, and I lay in the middle of an intersection completely knocked out. I woke up covered in blood, with a cracked skull and multiple broken bones. I picked myself up and started to stumble towards my apartment. I had no keys or phone and was unable to get in back inside so I decided to lay down in the grass and accept my fate. I closed my eyes and fell asleep. I woke up in a car rushing to the hospital, with my girlfriend at the time telling me everything was going to be okay. I spent a couple hours in the hospital where they cleaned and bandaged my wounds, gave me my painkillers and sent me on my way.

This time I knew I needed help but didn't know where to go. I called my parents, who said I could stay with them for a month in Tennessee under the agreement that I would find a job and a place to live during that time. I accepted their offer and flew to Portland to pick up their car to drive to Nashville, Tennessee. This is when I decided to cut myself off cold turkey. What better time to sober up than to drive cross country at 20 years old? I couldn't buy alcohol, and I didn't know anyone on the way to get any drugs from. It was the hardest drive of my life, and I had to face some real demons to get to Tennessee.

My addictions didn't stop there; they will always be a constant battle in my life, but I have learned moderation, and I've had a strong support system throughout my life. In both businesses that my wife and I have built, we've kept each other on the straight and narrow. My mother always gives me the confidence to push through the struggles in life and become a better person on the other side.

A Word from Kayla as Mom

The hardest thing I ever did was send Keegan to rehab. I wrestled with the decision, but ultimately, I knew that I would either be visiting my son's grave or visiting him in prison if I didn't grab for this last hope. The labor of motherhood does not end at delivery. It extends over a lifetime, and the dark years of Keegan's substance abuse disorder were the most painful years of my life. Staying sober during those years was a battle for me. After all, addiction is a distraction from what breaks us—and nothing broke me quite like the crushing worry for Keegan that consumed me day and night for years.

In those years, I wished for a *deus ex machine* known as a, "god from the machine" that is used as a fictional plot device in which a person or thing appears *out of the blue* to help a character to overcome a seemingly insolvable difficulty. But there was no *deus ex machine* for us. Getting and staying sober was only a decision that *only* Keegan could make. I had to decide for myself to stay sober and not escape into the bottle while Keegan wrested with his own substance abuse.

The week I sent Keegan to rehab I had a motivational blog post due for my business. I sat paralyzed, watching the blinking curser that seemed to mock me—you've failed, there is no hope, and a million other self-defeating messages. But eventually, I started to type and wrote "Narrate Me Down," which I would later read at Keegan's graduation from rehab and publish in my book *360 Degrees of Grief.* I hope it offers you some hope if you, as a parent or loved one of someone with substance abuse disorder, are in the midst of praying for your very own miracle or *deus ex machine.*

Narrate Me Down

I have a teenager. Enough said. End of sentence. No explanation needed. Everyone who has raised a teenager, everyone who is in the midst of raising a teenager and everyone who has ever been a teenager knows exactly what those words convey. There are moments of great pride and elation. Then there are days of despair, worry and angst.

In *The Many Adventures of Winnie the Pooh,* Tigger—having bounced himself up into a tree perfectly describes how I feel as a parent.

> **Narrator:** Well, Tigger, your bouncing really got you into trouble this time.
> **Tigger:** Say, who're you?
> **Narrator:** I'm the narrator.
> **Tigger:** Oh, well, please, for goodness sakes, narrate me down from here!
> **Narrator:** Very well. Hold on tight.[2]

In reality, my life goes on whether I am narrated out of the tree, or I climb down myself. I can't live life clinging to the tree. To say I have spent hours *on my knees* doesn't quite express the gravity of my prayers for my teenage son. I've found myself face first on the floor sucking carpet fibers while blowing snot bubbles in between weeping gasps over and over again lately. *Have you been there?* You know when you hear words that suddenly seize your strength, and you fall to the ground in despair. Maybe you are tougher than that, and you've been there, but you simply were braver than me, for I have spent these past few years intimately familiar with the deepest experiences of despair and hopelessness.

Some news hits you harder than others. In the depths of this grief, it is hard to imagine a day when this experience will have strengthened me. It was difficult to see the brightness of the future for any of us right now. I've wondered if, maybe, I would be granted a *deus ex machina* in which the ultimate Narrator would narrate us all down from this painful perch.

Life is full of ups and downs in which we all are looking around every corner for our very own *deus ex machina*. We have all read stories of restoration, recovery and hope. Some days when I am feeling blue, watching my heart walk outside of me in my teenage child, it is the hope of other people's stories that has lifted the suffocating elephant off of my chest.

On the really hard days when I was overwhelmed, I lean into what Christopher Robin said to Winnie the Pooh in the movie *Pooh's Grade Adventure*: "If there's ever a tomorrow when we're not together, there's something you should remember: You're braver than you believe, and stronger than you seem, and smarter than you think. But the most important thing is, even if we're apart, I'll always be with you."[3]

It is so true—even when Keegan and I were apart we were always together—tied together by the infinite love between a mother and her son. Today, we are all on the other side of these years. While Keegan was in rehab, I thought I was walking through the hardest years of my life. I missed him desperately. I would learn that his relapse years would be even harder. I worried every single time the phone rang that it would be a hospital or police department in Hawaii delivering the worst of news.

I wanted to speak words of wisdom that would redirect Keegan miraculously or even ground him for life, but he was an adult and all that I could do was love him right where he was— no matter what. I waited with open arms and with hopeful expectation. Finally, the waiting was rewarded when Keegan decided that he wanted more out of life. Today, we get to do life and business together. The awe of every moment of every day with my son is not lost on me.

If you are walking through addiction yourself, or coming along beside a loved one who is, I encourage you to never give up. Keep loving. Keep living. Keep trying, even when substance abuse wins a round—live for the next day with hopeful expectation.

Chapter 2
The Difference Between
Marijuana + Hemp

*"Then God said, 'I give you every seed-bearing plant on the face of
the whole earth and every tree that has fruit with seed in it.
They will be yours for food.'"*
Genesis 1:29 NIV

We believe it is important to know the difference between marijuana and hemp up front. Both marijuana and hemp come from the same species of plant, *Cannabis Sativa L.*, but that is where the similarities end. Hemp is cultivated differently and has completely different functions and applications. Hemp is said to have 25,000 uses. Marijuana has two—medical and recreational use.

The hemp plant contains a high level of cannabidiol (CBD) and only trace amounts of THC (regulated to 0.3%), while the marijuana plant has the opposite with a 5-30% THC content. THC is the psychoactive constituent of the *Cannibas* plant. Attempting to get high by smoking hemp would be a futile effort. Ministry of Hemp puts it this way, "Your lungs will fail before your brain attains any high from smoking industrial hemp."[1]

The hemp plant is the most misunderstood plant. David P. West Ph.D. captured it perfectly when he wrote, "Surely no member of the vegetable kingdom has ever been more misunderstood than hemp. For too many years, emotion—not reason—has guided our policy toward this crop. And nowhere have emotions run hotter than in the debate over the distinction between industrial hemp and marijuana."[2]

To break it down, hemp and marijuana are different varietals of the plant species *Cannabis.* One could say they are relatives, but scientifically opposites. By the legal definition, hemp contains a trace level of THC and a high level of CBD, while marijuana has low CBD and high THC. You can get high on marijuana, but you can't get high on hemp. Period.

Imagine for a moment that the poppy seed was as misunderstood as hemp. There are dozens of varieties of poppy flowers. The *Papaver somniferum* includes a variety of poppies known as the red scarlet, which produces opiates. The non-opium varieties of *Papaver somniferum* are completely legal to grow in your back yard despite the fact that the trace opiate level in the poppy seeds you buy for baking at the grocery store is actually higher than the trace THC level in hemp. Imagine if all poppy flowers had been banned because of the red scarlet variety. *There would be no lemon poppy seed muffins!*

According to Leaf Science, "The core agricultural differences between medical cannabis and hemp are largely in their genetic parentage and cultivation environment."[3] Hemp and marijuana are scientifically divergent and are cultivated in different ways. Hemp has completely different functions and applications than marijuana. For industrial hemp, the seeds, hurd and fiber are harvested. Hurd can be used for flooring, hempcrete and mulch. For marijuana, the flowering tops of the female plant, which are the source of Tetrahydrocannabinol (THC), are harvested. Hemp is an agricultural crop often referred to as industrial hemp. Marijuana is a horticultural crop.

Every part of the hemp plant has a use and potential market.

The oilseed of hemp is used in the cosmetic, soap, nutritional supplement and food industries. On multiple occasions, I have had people tell me that they took hemp oil, and it didn't help. When I asked further questions, I discovered that it was hemp seed oil that they were actually taking or rubbing on their body. Hemp seed oil and hemp CBD oil are two very different things. Hemp seed oil is lovely for a salad, but not quite the same thing at all.

Hemp seed oil is a rich source of essential omega-3 and omega-6 fatty acids, gamma-linolenic acid and proteins. It contains less than 10% saturated fats, and 70-80% polyunsaturated fatty acids. It is full of great stuff! Hemp seed oil does have a short shelf life and can quickly go rancid, which is an important reason not to use hemp seed oil to deliver hemp CBD oil.

When you buy hemp seed oil, it is recommended that you keep it in a refrigerator and make sure it is not exposed to light. It is sensitive to temperature fluctuation, so be sure to put it in the back of your fridge and not in the door. Hemp seed oil has many uses in the cosmetic and culinary industries. An unopened bottle of hemp seed oil that is *properly stored* can last as long as 12-14 months. However, once a bottle of hemp seed oil has been opened, it is recommended that it be consumed within 3-6 months.

The hemp plant has even more uses. The fiber and cellulose from hemp stalks are used in the textile, fuel and building industries. Hemp seed oil also has many household, industrial and technical uses. Hemp oilseed meal is used in animal feed, protein flours and powders. The hulled hemp seed is used in the food industry. The hemp stalk contains bast fibers and inner core. Bast fibers are one of the strongest plant fibers, which makes them a durable fiber for apparel, luggage, footwear and other textiles. Hemp bast fibers are used in the production of bio composites for household products, insulation, paper, packaging, clothing, bags, and can be used to replace plastics, fiberglass and wood. The hemp inner core of the stalk is used for animal bedding as a chemical absorbent that can be used after environmental spills, as well as can be used in farming and gardening. The whole hemp stalk can be used for biomass fuel. Hemp is the ultimate *green* product because it is renewable. Many products made with it are biodegradable and can be used to replace our dependence on non-renewable resources. The annual crop is great for farmers as a low-impact crop. Erik Rothenberg wrote, "These renewable resources will transition our major industries away from depending on non-renewable, fast-disappearing resource bases to being driven and supported on a sustainable economic basis by the annual agri-industrial produce of the Earth's fertile fields."[4]

Hemp CBD Oil

Hemp CBD oil is very different from hemp seed oil. The acronym CBD comes from the word cannabidiol, which is unique to the *Cannabis* plant. Cannabidiol interacts with the endocannabinoid system (ECS), which I will explain in great detail in chapter 4. Cannabinoids were first isolated by Roger Adams in 1940.[5]

Hemp CBD is often sold in three different forms. You will find references to full spectrum, broad spectrum and isolate. These are important distinctions. *Why?* One reason is that you rarely want to hear the words, "You're fired" from your employer. So, let's talk THC to make sure you make the right buying decisions when it comes to hemp CBD. Hemp CBD by legal definition can contain 0.3% or less THC as measured in the dried flowering portion of the plant. Drug tests for marijuana are pass/fail for the presence of THC. Since hemp CBD does contain 0.3% or less of THC, you can fail a drug test. In a 2018 story that hit the news in Tennessee, a woman took a drug test for a job promotion. Instead of being promoted, she was fired.[6]

If drug screening is part of your job requirements, you should be using a THC-free version of hemp CBD. When shopping for hemp CBD, if the packaging says *full spectrum*, that means the product does contain 0.3% or less of THC. If the product says *broad spectrum,* that means the cannabinoids of THC, THCV, and THCa have been lowered to parts per million, while leaving in the cannabinoids of CBD, CBN, CBDV, CBG, CBC, and CBN. If the product says *isolate,* that means the product was made from a single molecule 99%+ pure CBD without any other cannabinoids, terpenes, plant material, oil or chlorophyll.

What do you do if the product doesn't disclose whether it is THC-free or full spectrum? I suggest picking up another brand. This is basic information that should be fully disclosed.

Which version works better? The short answer is the one you can take! If having THC in a product makes it impossible for you to take hemp CBD, then the obvious choice is to choose an isolate or broad spectrum hemp CBD. You can't get the healing effect of Hemp CBD if you can't actually take it for one reason or another. Sometimes that comes down to the THC, and other times, it comes down to price. Products made with isolates are less expensive.

In theory, full spectrum has an entourage effect. Dr. Robert Pappas explains, "The entourage effect in the cannabis world usually refers to the enhanced effectiveness of the cannabinoids offered by the inclusion of the native terpenes of the plant. Some will also state it to more generally refer to the greater effectiveness of using the whole plant extract as opposed to just a single isolated cannabinoid"[7] (Dr. Robert Pappas 2018).

Chapter 3
Understanding Addiction

"The chains of habit are too weak to be felt until they are too strong to be broken." Samuel Johnson

Addiction. Addict. User. Alcoholic. Dopehead. Drug Abuser. Crackhead. Druggie. Junkie. Drunk. Pothead. These are all common words that are used in reference to people who struggle with substance abuse. Today, there is a movement to remove the stigma of addiction by changing the way we talk about it. The stigma, and a *fear of the stigma*, can cause people to avoid accepting that they have a substance abuse problem. In addition, we are more than our struggles with substance abuse. Instead, this movement is encouraging the use of the terms substance abuse disorder (SUD), in recovery, substance-free, alcohol and drug disorder and chemical dependency.

It is time to remove the stigma of someone becoming addicted to an addictive substance. According to the 2017 National Survey on Drug Use and Health, 19.7 million Americans age 12 or older had a substance use disorder.[1]

The perception that addiction is something that happens to someone else is best stated by Cathryn Kemp: "I used to think a drug addict was someone who lived on the far edges of society. Wild-eyed, shaven-headed and living in a filthy squat. That was until I became one..."[2]

Alcohol, nicotine, caffeine, many prescription and illicit

drugs are all addictive substances. It is no surprise that people become addicted to *addictive* substances when they use them. It does not make one person weaker than another. Addiction is a chronically relapsing disorder characterized by the compulsive desire to seek and use addictive substances.[3]

The neurotransmitter dopamine plays an important role in addiction. It is commonly referred to as the addiction molecule. In *This Naked Mind*, Annie Grace explains, "Addictive drugs, from nicotine to heroin, release artificially high levels of dopamine in the brain. While scientists used to believe dopamine was linked to feeling good, they now believe that dopamine is linked to learning, and learning includes wanting, expecting, and craving. Rather than giving us pleasure, dopamine teaches us how to get pleasure. It helps us learn the most effective ways to stimulate the brain's pleasure centers. We know that alcohol artificially stimulates the brain's pleasure centers. We also know that to maintain homeostasis and protect itself, the brain turns down the pleasure received from alcohol over time. Your brain is repeatedly over stimulated with alcohol, which builds a tolerance, the brain produces dynorphin to counter the over stimulation."[4] Dynorphin is an opioid peptide that promotes anxiety-like behavior and is associated with alcohol withdrawal.[5]

Basically, as we consume addictive substances, our brain adapts. Repeated and habitual use of addictive substances produces "incremental neuroadaptations in this neural system, rending it increasingly and perhaps permanently hypersensitive to the drug"[6] (Annie Grace 2018). This is why I (Kayla) haven't had a drink since 1992, because one glass of champagne at my graduation in 1990 brought me right back to full blown alcohol addiction for the next two years. The neuropathways of my brain are permanently changed to create an additive response to alcohol for the rest of my life.

When you are addicted to a substance, there can be significant negative consequences to the addict and the people connected to them. Becoming dependent on a substance creates a physical and psychological cycle of abuse, dependence and craving. The body experiences withdrawal from the addictive substance, which makes the person suffering from a chemical dependency crave the substance on a daily basis. Annie Grace says it best in relation to alcohol abuse: "What is important now is to realize that alcohol does pick you up, but only from how far it kicked you down, never up to where you were before you started drinking"[7] (Grace 2018).

Addictive substances release artificially high levels of dopamine in the brain. As I mentioned scientists now know that dopamine is not linked to feeling good, but instead is linked to learning—learning how to get pleasure repeatedly by creating wanting, expectation and craving for the substance. And with repeated use, this creates tolerance. Once tolerance is created, you need more and more of the same substance to get the pleasure it once brought.

Next, withdrawal creates unpleasant symptoms when you stop taking the substance because your brain has changed to compensate for the chronic presence of the substance. Once the abuse, tolerance and withdrawal cycle are in full swing, extremely strong and illogical cravings complete the cycle of addiction[8] (Annie Grace 2018).

To get technical, addictive substances increase cravings by releasing artificially high levels of dopamine. As part of the reward circuit, this results in an increased dopamine level in nucleus accumbens, part of the basal forebrain. In the addictive cycle, the increased levels of dopamine create compulsive and illogical cravings. Eventually the brain compensates for this over stimulation by numbing the pleasure center.[9]

There is no cure for addiction. There are, however, ways that hemp CBD can help with the withdrawal symptoms associated with addiction. There isn't a miracle cure that will take away the cycle of abuse, dependence and craving, but research is showing that hemp CBD can bring some assistance to the person who wishes to break the addiction cycle.

Most importantly for anyone who suffers from substance abuse issues is whether or not hemp CBD is in-and-of-itself an addictive substance. The short answer is that it is not. The key to understanding why hemp CBD is not an additive substance is the fact that it does not release excessive levels of dopamine into the brain. Instead of getting you high, hemp CBD works to create a balanced level of neurotransmitter into the brain— or homeostasis.

For anyone, like me (Kayla), who wants to be extra cautious, it is important that we talk about the 0.3% or less THC that is legally present in full spectrum hemp CBD products. THC does create a high and does release dopamine in the brain. However, the antagonistic properties of CBD counteract the psychoactive properties of the level of THC found in hemp.

Chapter 4
Cannabidiol +
the Endocannabinoid System

"You are the most awesome living organism on the plant. Your mind can do more than any computer. In fact, it creates computers. Your body is self-regulating, self-healing, and self-aware. It alerts you to the tiniest problems and is programmed to protect you, ensuring your survival. It is infinitely more complex than the most intelligent technology. It is priceless."[1]
Annie Grace from This Naked Mind

The endocannabinoid system plays an important role in the overall health of someone struggling with substance abuse by maintaining and establishing homeostasis. Generally, we are taught about just a handful of the systems of the human body. Most people are not aware there is also the endocannabinoid system. Cannabidiol (CBD) interacts with the endocannabinoid system (ECS). The acronym CBD comes from the word cannabidiol, a compound unique to the *cannabis* plant, which produces phyto-cannabinoids. The ECS is made up of cannabinoid receptors, endocannabinoids, and the enzymes that break down endocannabinoids. The ECS is made up of millions of cannabinoid receptor sites (CB1 and CB2) that are throughout our entire body, including our nervous system, skin, immune cells in our bloodstream and our brain—even hair follicles and mast cells, and so much more. The human body always seeks to maintain homeostasis, or more easily stated, to balance bodily functions. The endocannabinoid system maintains equilibrium in the body by seeking to correct anything that gets out of balance, including mood, sleep, hormones, fertility, memory, energy, anxiety, immune response, appetite, pain and more. Dr. Dustin Sulak states, "In each tissue, the endocannabinoid system performs different tasks, but the goal is always the same: homeostasis, the maintenance of a stable internal environment despite fluctuations in the external environment"[2] (Dr. Dustin Sulak).

What is so important about homeostasis? *Health. Survival. Wellness.* "Homeostasis, from the Greek words for 'same' and 'steady,' refers to any process that living things use to actively maintain fairly stable conditions necessary for survival"[3] (Kevin Rodolfo 2000).

Even though the human body produces cannabinoid, it is possible to have cannabinoid deficiency. In a study on PubMed, E.B. Russo explains, "Migraine, fibromyalgia, IBS and related conditions display common clinical, biochemical and pathophysiological patterns that suggest an underlying clinical endocannabinoid deficiency that may be suitably treated with cannabinoid medicines"[4] (E.B. Russo 2004). The average American diet has not contained cannabinoids, until recently with the rise of Hemp CBD oil, which contains cannabidiol as well as over 85 other cannabinoids. The plant genus *Cannabis* is the only source, outside the human body, that produces cannabinoids.

Cannabinoids are divided into two groups:
1. Endocannabinoids, which are produced naturally by the endocannabinoid system.
2. Phyto-cannabinoids, which are found in the *Cannabis*

plant. When talking about hemp CBD, we are referring to phyto-cannabinoids.

Addiction puts the entire body at risk. There is no body system that is immune to the ravages of drug and alcohol abuse. To better understand the job of the endocannabinoid system, it is important to quickly review the other body systems that it helps regulate. None of the body systems operate independently—what damages one, damages many.

Cardiovascular System includes the heart, blood and vessels (veins, arteries and capillaries). Excessive alcohol use causes cardiovascular risks and disorder, including heart damage, irregular heartbeat, stroke, high blood pressure, weakening of the heart muscle, higher level of triglycerides, increased caloric intake and sudden cardiac death.[5] Drugs have an adverse impact on the cardiovascular system, including cocaine, heroin, marijuana, methamphetamine, prescriptions, steroids, synthetic cannabinoids and tobacco.[6]

Respiratory System includes the nose, trachea, lungs and rib muscles. Tobacco products have a well-known negative impact on the respiratory system. According to the American Addiction Centers, "So-called 'smoker's cough' is often a result of the lungs attempting to rid themselves of impurities associated with tobacco products. Over time, these products take their toll, and many of the carcinogens cannot be removed completely…Toxic chemicals in cigarettes and other tobacco products number literally in the hundreds, and eventually, these substances lead to an increase in the risk of getting certain respiratory conditions and the risk of developing numerous forms of cancer by changing the cellular structure of the tissues."[7] In addition to the higher risk of cancer, tobacco products put consumers at a high risk for COPD, asthma and lung infections.

Opioids and cocaine worsen existing respiratory disorders and cause significant risk for pulmonary edema. Cocaine can also cause ruptures in the air sacs of the lungs. Those who snort cocaine are at a higher risk of damage to the trachea and nasal passages. As a central nervous system depressant, alcohol reduces the breathing rate of people who drink.[8]

The jury is still out on whether or not smoking marijuana increases risks to the respiratory system—however many conclusively have determined that the risks are lower than smoking tobacco. However, the use of vape products for nicotine, CBD, and THC are not safe. A hot topic of debate in the hemp CBD industry is vaping. Our company has made a firm stance to be on the right side of history of the vaping craze—so we do not sell vape products. Our lungs were not designed to process chemicals, flavoring chemicals, propylene glycol, polyethylene glycol, toxic chemicals used to adulterate or lipids such as fractionated coconut oil, petroleum products or hemp seed oil. There are some reports of hospitalizations caused by CBD vape products that actually contained synthetic marijuana, also known as K2, Spice or AK47.

Skeletal System includes bones and joints. One might think that drinking alcohol would not impact your skeletal system, but it does. In an article on WebMD, Dr. Primal Kaur explains, "Alcohol interferes with the pancreas and its absorption of calcium and vitamin D. Alcohol also affects the liver, which is important for activating vitamin D—which is also important for calcium absorption. The hormones important to bone health also go awry. Some studies suggest that alcohol decreases estrogen and can lead to irregular periods. As estrogen declines, bone remodeling slows and leads to bone loss. If you're in the menopausal years, this adds to the bone loss that's naturally occurring. There's an increase in two potentially bone-damaging hormones, cortisol and parathyroid hormone. High levels of cortisol seen in people with alcoholism can decrease bone formation and increase bone breakdown. Chronic alcohol consumption also increases parathyroid hormone, which leaches calcium from the bone" (Jeanie Lerche Davis).[9] The use of other drugs can cause the same lack of nutrient metabolism. All intoxication increases the risks of falls from inebriation and injuries caused by poor judgement decision making caused by lower inhibitions.

Urinary System includes the bladder, kidneys, ureters and the urethra. Excessive drinking directly damages the renal system. Also, the liver and kidneys work together so the damage alcohol causes to the liver impacts kidney function. Excessive alcohol consumption depletes minerals, creates an electrolyte imbalance and alters the acidity levels in the renal system. Nicotine is a toxic substance which increases the rate of kidney disease, increases the level of albumin, narrows the renal arteries, inflames the kidneys and disrupts the balance of fluids and electrolytes in the renal system. Other drugs have significant negative impacts on the kidneys. One-third of cocaine users who are admitted into the emergency room develop acute kidney disease.[10]

Muscular System includes the muscles and tendons. Chronic alcohol use can lead to muscle weakness, cramping and atrophy, but also to a condition known as rhabdomyolysis, which causes muscle tissue to break down, which causes the release of toxins in the bloodstream, eventually leading to kidney failure and a compromised muscular system. Ironically, opiate drugs used commonly to reduce pain actually cause an increase in muscle aches and pain.[11]

Endocrine System includes glands and hormones. Even the moderate use of alcohol can increase the risk of hormone-receptor-positive breast cancer in women.[12] Heavy drinking can cause hypoglycemia and lead to osteoporosis by interfering with the way the endocrine system absorbs calcium. In men, heavy drinking can cause a loss of testosterone, which can result in shrinking testicles, low semen count, emotional issues, breast growth and erectile dysfunction.[13] Opioids can cause loss of sex drive, irregular menstrual cycles and risk for osteoporosis.[14]

Digestive System includes the mouth, esophagus, stomach, intestines, throat, liver, gall bladder, pancreas, rectum and anus. When alcohol is metabolized, the body creates a toxic substance known as acetaldehyde, which has been found to be mutagenic and carcinogenic. Acetaldehyde wreaks havoc in the human body—so much so that it was hard to decide which body system to place it under, but it is the liver where an enzyme known as alcohol dehydrogenase (ADH) transforms alcohol into acetaldehyde.[15]

Anyone who has had too many drinks is mostly already aware that alcohol irritates the digestive system. There is nothing glamorous about bowing down to the porcelain god. In addition, alcohol damages the lining and muscles of your stomach and esophagus. "In 2012, the International Cancer Research Agency assessed ethanol as a group 1 carcinogen in alcoholic beverages. While alcohol is a contributing cause of liver and breast cancer, your digestive system allows for heavy consumption of alcohol that can increase risks of mouth, throat, and bowel cancer as well as colon and rectum...Four or more drinks a day significantly increases the chances of gastrointestinal cancer development"[16](Brandon Shavers 2019).

Opioid drugs can cause constipation, acid reflux and abdominal pain. Cocaine impairs tissues in the bowels. Nicotine is related to colon, esophagus and stomach cancers. And according to a paper published in the journal *Acta Chirurgica Iugoslavica,* drug use in general can cause rectal bleeding, ischemic colitis and long-term damage to the colon.[17]

Nervous System includes the brain, spinal cord and nerves. Alcohol is a depressant to the nervous system, which in the short-term impacts vision, judgment and decision making, reaction time, coordination and alertness. Chronic long term alcohol use can also cause some of these symptoms (and more) to be permanent, including memory loss, confusion, behavior changes, balance and coordination problems and peripheral neuropathy, which causes damage to the nerves in your feet and hands.[18] Too much alcohol can actually cause the cells in your brain to shrink. Mind-altering drugs can slow down or speed up the central nervous systems and autonomic functions. In later chapters, we will go into more depth about how drugs disrupt neurotransmitters, but it is important to note that drugs can affect dopamine, serotonin, gamma-aminobutyric acid (GABA) and norepinephrine.[19]

Lymphatic System includes the lymph, lymph nodes, lymphatic vessels, lymphatic capillaries and the spleen. Chronic use of drugs and alcohol can cause scarring in the venous and lymphatic system, which can lead to lymphedema, an accumulation of fluid in the lymph nodes. Lymphedema can increase the risk of infections and diseases. Cancers caused by excessive alcohol and drug use can also block the lymphatic ducts.[20]

Integumentary System includes the epidermis, dermis, hydro-dermis, hair follicles, sweat pores, sweat glands, oil glands and sensory receptors. The skin is greatly impacted by what we put in our bodies. In most cases, the negative response will be inflammation and immune reactions. In the short-term, dehydration can cause the skin to appear dull, in the long-term chronic dehydration causes wrinkles. Alcohol dehydrates your system. Chronic inflammation caused by long term drinking causes a release of histamine that dilates the capillaries, which can result in skin redness and spider-like veins known as spider angioma. In the short term, alcohol also dilates the pores, which can cause blackheads and whiteheads[21] (Adam Hurly 2017).

Drug abuse can cause a variety of skin infections, ulcers, sores and inflammation, and can even cause rotting of the skin caused by skin cell death known as necrosis. Meth is infamous for 'meth mites,' which is actually a false sensation of insects crawling on or under their skin, resulting in chronic picking of the skin.[22]

Olfactory System includes specialized sensory cells known as olfactory sensory neurons, which send messages to your brain. Excessive alcohol use can lead to deficits in the sense of smell that new studies are finding have found are linked to frontal lobe damage caused by chronic alcohol consumption. Claudia I. Rupp, clinical neuropsychologist and assistant professor in the department of psychiatry at Innsbruck Medical University states, "Olfactory dysfunction can seriously impair people in their day-to-day activities and occupation, increase their risk of injury or even death, and reduce their overall quality of life. These deficits may not only reduce patients' enjoyment of foods but may also place them at risk for long term nutritional or health sequelae. Individuals may alter food choices and intake, resulting in weight loss, challenged immunity and impaired nutritional status...all of which are commonly observed in patients with chronic alcoholism."[22]

Auditory System is the sensory system for the sense of hearing, which includes the peripheral auditory system and the central auditory system. Anyone who has had too much to drink has experience the dizziness caused by the change in the volume and composition of the fluid in the inner ear. Long term excessive alcohol use can cause hearing loss. Even after alcohol has left your blood stream and brain, it is still present in the fluid of your inner ear.[23] Excessive alcohol use damages the auditory cortex in your brain. Also, the toxic environment caused by alcohol damages the tiny hair cells that are designed to send auditory messages to the brain. Alcohol can also cause long term tinnitus.[24]

In 2001 Rush Limbaugh's hearing loss was all over the news as it was linked to his addiction to painkillers. It remains up for debate whether his hearing loss was caused by painkillers. Dr. Jeffery Harris explained, "It's pretty clear that there is this association. The ear is sensitive to drugs, and this particular association with Vicodin has become more relevant as people are getting their hands on it as a recreational drug."[25]

Immune System includes a network of cells, tissues and organs that work together to respond to *foreign* invaders, such as bacteria, parasites, viruses and fungi. White blood cells (leukocytes) circulate in the body between organs and lymph nodes via lymphatic vessels and blood vessels. Leukocytes can be either *phagocytes,* which are cells that chew up invading organisms, or *lymphocytes,* which are cells that allow the body to recall and recognize previous *foreign* invaders. This helps the body to destroy returning invaders.

Excessive alcohol consumption leads to immunodeficiency, resulting in increased infectious diseases. Organ damage, especially to the liver, may be partially caused by alcohol-triggered autoimmunity, an immune response of the body against healthy cells and tissues. Alcoholics are twice as likely to die of pneumonia.[26] The damage excessive alcohol does to the cardiovascular system, liver, digestive system, respiratory and more increases the impact of alcohol on the immune system. Excessive drinking damages the macrophages and T and C cells in your immune system, which overall, weakens the immune system. Drug users are more likely to contract hepatitis, sexually transmitted diseases and HIV. Prescription opioids surpass the immune system through a brain-to-body pathway, which eventually leads to the suppression of white blood cells.[27]

Reproductive System includes internal and external organs involved in procreation. The male reproductive system includes the testes and the penis. The female reproductive system can be divided into internal and external structures. The female external structures include the clitoris, labia minora, labia majora and Bartholin's glands. The internal female structures include the vagina, uterus, ovaries, cervix and fallopian tubes.

Excessive alcohol impacts the male reproductive system by causing reduced testosterone levels, which can lead to shrunken testes, infertility, impotence, breast enlargement, as well as reduced chest and facial hair. In males, alcohol can affect how hormones from the pituitary and hypothalamus glands are released. Excessive drinking in females can cause disruption in menstrual cycles, increased risk of miscarriage, early menopause and increased risk of breast cancer.[28]

Endocannabinoid System (ECS) is a complete cell-signaling system. Raphael Mechoulam at Hebrew University in Jerusalem became the first to isolate THC in 1964. Lumír Hanuš and William Devane, who worked on Raphael Mechoulam's team, isolated the first known endocannabinoid, anandamine (AEA), in the human brain on March 24, 1992. This discovery confirmed that the human brain produces cannabinoids.[29] Raphael Mechoulam and Shimon Ben-Shabat discovered the endocannabinoid 2-Arachidonoylglycerol (2-AG).

The human body has both CB1 and CB2 receptors. CB1 receptors are mostly found in the central nervous system. CB2 receptors are mostly in your peripheral nervous system. Both endocannabinoids and phyto-cannabinoids can bind to either CB1 or CB2 receptors. Once endocannabinoids have done their job, the two different enzymes break them down. The enzyme fatty acid amide hydrolase breaks down anandamine (AEA), and monoacylglycerol acid lipase breaks down 2-Arachidonoylglycerol (2-AG). The cannabinoid THC also interacts with the endocannabinoid system and can bind to both CB1 and CB2 receptors, but the high from THC comes from it binding to CB1 receptors.[30]

A study by Laprairie et al found that CBD acts as a non-competitive negative allosteric modulator of CB1 receptors, which means that CBD decreases agonist binding or receptor signaling of THC. CBD, as an allosteric modulator of the CB1 receptor, allows the cannabinoids to still treat disorders of the central and peripheral systems while blocking any adverse reactions of THC, such as paranoia, while leaving intact the positive properties, such as anti-nausea and analgesic effects. It is believed that CBD prevents endocannabinoids from being broken down, allowing for better use and distribution. It is also possible that there are more receptors that have not been discovered yet.[31]

Given all the damage that excessive alcohol use, and in some cases even moderate use (as well as drug abuse), inflicts on the body, the endocannabinoid system has its work cut out for it. The endocannabinoid system shows great promise as a therapeutic tool in the addiction cycle because, "Endocannabinoids themselves function as neuromodulators that are released by post-synaptic neurons, and bind to the presynaptic CB1Rs to moderate the release of neurotransmitters, such as gamma-aminobutyric-acid (GABA), glutamate, and dopamine. While the specific CB1R function depends on the cell population and region in which they reside, their role in retrograde signaling permits them to regulate signaling activity across cognitive, emotive, and sensory functions, lending therapeutic capacity"[32] (Yann Chye et al 2019).

Dr. Melanie Bone, a cannabis physician and gynaecologist, states, "Utilization of the ECS as part of an integrative approach to managing addiction and its consequences, has great potential. I believe that a successful, long term approach to addiction should involve optimizing the ECS along with other treatment modalities such as therapy, support groups, and allopathic medications. What this may consist of is supplementation with hemp CBD products to help stabilize the neurological component of addiction. This alone will not be sufficient and it must be implemented along with lifestyle changes and regular counseling to ensure ongoing support that is at the heart of successful sobriety"[33] (Dr. Bone, personal communication, November 3, 2019).

Chapter 5
Hemp CBD + Alcohol Addiction

"First you take a drink, then the drink takes a drink,
then the drink takes you." F. Scott Fitzgerald

Recently a Facebook post from the page *Her View from Her Home* stated, "Being alcohol free can truly feel ostracizing. And it's strange to think that alcohol is the only drug that we have to explain NOT using." I shared her story and added, "Personally, I'm happy to be along whether people are drinking or not—but I know some people aren't comfortable with me not drinking with them. I have no problem telling people I'm an alcoholic— I feel no shame in being sober or for the years I lost to alcohol—but I know many don't like being forced to explain their abstinence from alcohol, whatever their personal reason is."[1]

Alcohol is a drug. It is classified as a depressant—it slows down the vital functions in your body. With two or more drinks, it acts as a stimulant, and beyond that, alcohol acts as a depressant. The more you drink—the closer you are to death as your vital functions diminish. Alcoholism often starts so slowly that people miss the fact that they have a substance abuse problem. Alcohol is slow to kill, but it is insidious and hideous in how it destroys your body.[2]

According to BreastCancer.org, women who drink beer, wine and liquor have an increased risk of hormone-receptor-positive breast cancer because alcohol damages DNA cells and increases the levels of estrogen and other hormones related to hormone-receptor-positive breast cancer. "Compared to women who don't drink at all, women who have three alcoholic drinks per week have a 15% higher risk of breast cancer. Experts estimate that the risk of breast cancer goes up another 10% for each additional drink women regularly have each day."[3]

In *This Naked Truth* Annie Grace wrote, "Alcohol is society's most dangerous addiction, causing four times as many deaths as prescription and illegal drug overdoses combined. And it's growing. Death by alcohol consumption is increasing every year, and it has now surpassed AIDS as the world's number one killer of men aged 15-59. More people are addicted to alcohol than any other drug on the planet. Yet we've stigmatized not drinking"[4] (Annie Grace 2018).

Alcohol is an addictive substance. And only caffeine and alcohol are socially acceptable addictive substances. Annie Grace wrote, "...consider the possibility that since we are human, and since alcohol is addictive to humans, once we begin to drink, we unconsciously begin a slow slide into addiction"[5] (Annie Grace 2018).

A study in *JAMA Psychiatry* journal found that one in eight American adults meets the criteria for alcohol disorder.[6] (The DSM-5 criteria can be found in the resources section in the back of the book.) It may seem that alcohol abuse doesn't do the kind of damage as addiction to something like heroin. However, this was disproven by a study done on behalf of the Independent Scientific Committee on Drugs in 2010. This study analysed the social, physical and psychological harm to those abusing alcohol and the people in their lives. The impact was scored on a scale of 0 (for the no harm) to 100 (for the highest harm). The drugs with the highest total harm-score to the user were heroin (34), crack cocaine (37) and methamphetamine (32). The drugs with the highest total harm-score to others were alcohol (42), crack cocaine (17) and heroin (21). However, when the harm-scores to the user and to others in their lives were combined, alcohol had the highest-harm score (72), followed by heroin (55), and crack cocaine (54)[7] (Professor David J. Nutt et al 2010).

According to the National Institute on Alcohol Abuse and Alcoholism, every year an estimated 88,000 people die from alcohol-related diseases.[8] That means that alcohol accounts for nearly double the total number of people who die of drug-induced causes in the United States.[9] The National Institute on Drug Abuse reports that over 23% of admissions into public health treatment centers are for alcohol abuse.[10]

The symptoms of alcohol withdrawal include anxiety, irritability, headache, sleep disorders, tremors, sweating, nausea and hallucinations. Using hemp CBD while consuming alcohol and/or while attempting to withdraw from the use of alcohol can help with these symptoms.

Studies have found that hemp CBD can help the body recover from the damage done to the brain by excessive alcohol. What is incredibly promising is that the studies done with rats in relation to alcohol addiction are based on topical application of CBD. In one study, rats with a history of self-administration of alcohol were given transdermal CBD at 24-hour intervals for seven days. The rats were tested for context (starting point and triggers), stress-induced reinstatement (drug relapse and craving are often provoked by stress) and anxiety. Topical application of hemp CBD reduced drug seeking behaviour, reduced anxiety and prevented the development of high impulsivity in the rats with alcohol dependence without causing any sedative effect or reducing motivation. What is even more interesting is that even after the treatment of topical CBD was terminated, the effects remained for approximately 5 months, despite the fact that the CBD was only detectable for 3 days after treatment was ceased[11] (Gonzalez-Cuevas et al 2018).

The long-lasting impact of hemp CBD in this study is incredibly promising. The neuroprotective properties of hemp CBD are on display with these results. Excessive alcohol consumption results in neurodegeneration and behavioral and cognitive impairments. The fact that the rats had the same results 5 months after application as they did during the study shows that even topical CBD can improve damage done from excessive alcohol consumption.

A study by Daniel J. Liput et al used transdermal gel at 1.0%, 2.5% and 5.0% of CBD to treat alcohol-induced neurodegeneration. The study found that the 5.0% CBD gel resulted in a 48.8% reduction in neurodegeneration in the entorhinal cortex. A second experiment used a 2.5% CBD gel and compared the results to a CBD intraperitoneal injection (injection into the peritoneum, a.k.a. body cavity) at a dose of 40mg/kg per day. The second experiment found that both routes of administration provided similar neuroprotection results. The 2.5% CBD gel resulted in a 56.1% reduction in neurodegeneration, while the injection resulted in a 50.6% reduction[12] (Daniel J. Liput et al 2013).

Despite the damage excessive drinking does to our body, the cycle of addiction is illogical. In *This Naked Mind*, Annie Grace explains,

Since alcohol takes up to ten days to leave your body, the lows can be ever-present for regular drinkers. It is not that alcohol makes you happy. It's that as a drinker, you are unhappy when you are unable to drink. Scratching an itch is pleasurable, but you would never purposely sit in poison ivy just to scratch your ass. This is a key to all drug addiction—the drug creates the low and then deceives its victim into believing that, by ending the low, it is providing a high.

That's how drugs work, and the further they take you down, the greater your perceived need becomes. With alcohol it can be so gradual you barely notice you are falling. As you drink, your tolerance grows, and soon you need to drink more to get the same effects. It can happen quickly, but often it happens slowly, over a lifetime[13] (Annie Grace 2018).

It is promising to find that CBD helps protect your brain against the damage of alcohol. Alcohol causes inflammation and damage throughout your entire body but is especially damaging to the liver and brain. Excessive alcohol slowly kills off the neurons in our brain. This neurodegeneration is considered a main component of alcohol abuse disorders.

Alcohol has been found to have a downstream potentiation effect on the endocannabinoid system in rats. The levels of anandamide and 2-AG are increased with use of alcohol, while the cannabinoid receptor type 1 are decreased. It is thought that the disruption of endocannabinoid signaling may prove effective in treating substance abuse disorders.[14] Other potential benefits of hemp CBD in addiction are the anti-anxiety, stress-reducing, anti-depressant and anti-compulsive properties.

Chapter 6
Hemp CBD + Nicotine Addiction

"People always come up to me and say that my smoking is bothering them...Well, it's killing me!" Wendy Liebman

Approximately 50 million Americans are addicted to tobacco products, including cigarettes, cigars, chewing tobacco and snuff.[1] The use of e-cigarettes is on the rise as well. Many believe that e-cigarette users are transitioning away from traditional tobacco products, however analysis in the *Annals of Internal Medicine* estimates that 1.9 million American adults who currently vape never smoked cigarettes[2] (Daniel Allar 2018).

Nicotine temporarily stimulates dopamine production and creates a sense of euphoria or pleasure. It also stimulates the adrenal glands, which causes the blood pressure and heart rate to rise. Nicotine binds to the nicotinic cholinergic receptors. These receptors adapt to nicotine, and eventually, the brain needs more nicotine for the same impact.

A study by Morgan et al found that CBD reduced cigarette consumption in tobacco smokers. The study was a randomized, double-blind, placebo-controlled study of 24 smokers who wanted to reduce smoking. Of the group, 12 were given a CBD inhaler, and 12 were given a placebo to use for one week with the instruction to use the inhaler whenever they felt the urge to smoke. The placebo group showed no reduction in cigarette use. The group given the inhaler with CBD reduced the number of cigarettes they smoked during the treatment week by 40%[3] (C.J. Morgan et al 2013).

A study by Hindocha et al asked 30 smokers to abstain from tobacco use overnight, after which the researchers gave the participants either 800 mg of internal CBD or a placebo. The researchers wanted to determine whether CBD would reduce cravings. The participants were shown images related to smoking in an effort to induce cravings. The CBD group had reduced perceived pleasure from these images compared to the placebo group. Neither group had a significant reduction in cravings[4] (Hidocha et al).

A study by Chye et al states, "Nicotine activates DA (dopaminergic) neurons in the VTA (ventral tegmental area) either directly through stimulation of nicotinic cholinergic receptors or indirectly through glutaminergic nerve terminals that are modulated by the ECS (endocannabinoid system)"[41] (Chye et al).

Quitting the habit of smoking causes not only withdrawal, but anxiety. CBD has been shown to have anti-anxiety properties that we will discuss in further detail in Chapter 13.

Chapter 7
Hemp CBD + Opioid Addiction

"If you can quit for a day, you can quit for a lifetime."
Benjamin Alire Sáenz

According to the National Institute on Drug Abuse as of January 2019, 130 people die every day from an opioid overdose. Opioids include prescription pain relievers, heroin and synthetic opioids, such as fentanyl. The genesis of the opioid crisis was in the late 1990's when pharmaceutical companies claimed that prescription opioid pain relievers were not addictive.

Fast forward to 2019 and those same drug companies are being sued to help pay for the crisis they created. In September of 2019, Purdue Pharma, the makers of OxyContin, have tentatively agreed to pay as much as $12 billion to settle lawsuits—which in our opinion is nothing in comparison to the over 700,000 overdose deaths related to it since 1999. The legal linchpin of these cases, and the many more to come, is that the drug companies knew, or should have known, that their products weren't safe, and yet they advertised their drugs as safe and effective anyway.

The reality was that 21-29% of patients prescribed opioids for chronic pain misused them. Of those, 8-12% developed an opioid use disorder, and 4-6% of those with opioid use disorder transferred their addiction to heroin. Furthermore,

80% of heroin users first misused a prescription opioid.[1] This move to heroin wasn't generally because patients who were prescribed opioids wanted a better high, but because the high cost of opioids, and the obstacles in place to block misuse of them, made it hard to obtain legal prescriptions—yet the pain persisted for these patients. The risk of taking heroin in place of opioids is high. Heroin is often laced with fentanyl.

Opioid withdrawal symptoms include: flu-like symptoms, fever, sweating, dilated pupils, runny nose and eyes, body aches, anxiety, insomnia, as well as nausea, vomiting or diarrhea. Drug relapse from opioid use disorder (OUD) is exceptionally high. Abstinence-based protocols have resulted in 85% relapse within one year, and in-patient programs, have an 80% relapse history within two years. Patients using abstinence, plus an opioid replacement such as methadone, resulted in 40% relapse within in the first year. Evidence shows that medication-assisted pharmacotherapy, combined with social support, is the most effective tool to preventing relapse. New early research shows that hemp CBD can be useful in the reduction of withdrawal symptoms, since CBD has been shown to have anti-anxiety, anti-psychotic, antidepressant and neuroprotective properties. According to Wiese and Wilson-Poe, "Numerous pre-clinical studies have shown that cannabis and cannabinoids decrease opioid withdrawal symptoms"[2] (Wiese and Wilson Poe 2018).

A study by Katsidoni, Anagnostou and Panagis suggests that CBD interferes with brain reward mechanisms that are responsible for the expression of the acute reinforcing properties of opioids, which indicates that CBD may be useful in reducing the reward effects of opioids. They found that CBD has an impact on the both the intoxication and relapse phases of opioid addiction[3] (Katsidoni, Anagnostou, and Panagis 2013).

A study by Ren et al found that CBD reduced heroin-seeking behavior anywhere from 24 hours to two weeks, which suggests that CBD may be a potential treatment for heroin craving and relapse[4] (Ren et al 2009).

In the article "Can CBD Treat Opioid Addiction," Dr. Shereef Elnahal, commissioner of New Jersey's Department of Health, said, "CBD has promising effects on pain, which could make it an effective substitute for opioids."[5] In an investigation by the JAMA Network, they found, "This longitudinal analysis of Medicare Part D found that prescriptions filled for all opioids decreased by 2.11 million daily doses per year from an average of 23.08 million daily doses per year when a state instituted any medical cannabis law. Prescriptions for all opioids decreased by 3.742 million daily doses per year when medical cannabis dispensaries opened."[6]

A Consumer Reports article quoted Dr. Howard Zucker, the New York State Health Commissioner, who said, "Adding opioid replacement as a qualifying condition for medical marijuana offers providers another treatment option, which is a critical step in combating the deadly opioid epidemic"[7] (Rachel Rabkin Peachman 2019). The good news is that hemp CBD is legal in most states and is effective in the treatment of pain and inflammation.

A review by Wiese and Wilson-Poe in "Cannabis and Cannabinoid Research" stated that, "The endocannabinoid and opioidergic systems are known to interact in many different ways, from the distribution of their receptors to cross-sensitization of their behavioral pharmacology. Cannabinoid-1 (CB1) receptors and mu opioid receptors (MORs) are distributed in many of the same areas in the brain...The extent of this overlapping expression and frequent co-localization of the CB1 and MOR provide clear morphological underpinnings for interactions between the opioid and cannabinoid systems in reward and withdrawal"[8] (Wiese and Wilson-Poe).

The primary reason for opioid prescriptions is for the analgesic properties.

Dr. Bone, who is a cannabis physician and gynaecologist, says, "Opiates, when utilized appropriately, offer a low-cost and highly efficacious approach to both acute and chronic pain. We need to view CBD and other cannabis products as another tool in our shed to aid in preventing inappropriate utilization of opiates. As a practicing medical cannabis provider, I see that the addition of cannabinoids to the treatment plan, results in spontaneous reduction in opiate use. On the other hand, it is uncommon for CBD or other cannabinoids to completely replace opiates. The two products work on different receptors and often potentiate the effects of one another.

Also, on a more practical note, the cost factor is key. Opiates cost a fraction of cannabinoids. Lastly, the aging demographic is accustomed to picking up a medication at the pharmacy with a co-pay. These people find the lack of authoritative guidance about CBD or other cannabinoids and the difficulty in obtaining a medical card in many states as a daunting roadblock to trying it. Fear of unknown reactions, medication interactions, and risk, all play a part in this perception. They are more comfortable with what they are accustomed to using and feeling, and therefore adopting a new approach seems overwhelming to them.

Lastly, we don't have long term longitudinal evidence of safety and efficacy to substantiate it"[9] (Bone 2019).

Chapter 8
Hemp CBD
+ Marijuana Addiction

*"The chains of habit are weak to be felt until they
are too strong to be broken." Samuel Johnson*

Some believe that you can't get addicted to marijuana, however
recent data suggests that 30% of marijuana users have some
degree of marijuana dependence disorder[1] (Hasin et al 2015).
Research done by the University College of London has found
that marijuana users that *skunk* cannabis (a.k.a. *skunk* weed) are
more likely to develop cannabis dependence.[2] The term *skunk
cannabis* comes from old-school popular marijuana that has a
skunky or stinky aroma.

According to the National Institute of Drug Abuse,
"Marijuana dependence occurs when the brain adapts to large
amounts of the drug by reducing production of and sensitivity
to its own endocannabinoid neurotransmitters."[3]

A study of active marijuana users found that isolated CBD
did not show any potential of addiction[5] (Babalonis et al 2017).
This is important for those concerned that they may be trading
one addiction for another.

In a case study, a 19-year-old woman who was suffering
from cannabis withdrawal syndrome was treated with CBD
(300 mg on the first day, 600 mg on days 2-10 and 300 mg on
day 11) for a total of 11 days. What researchers found when

they took daily assessments was that she was not experiencing significant withdrawal, anxiety or dissociative symptoms. They concluded that CBD was effective for the treatment of cannabis withdrawal[4] (Crippa et al 2013).

In a 2011 research case at the Wholeness Center, a 27-year-old male with bipolar depression and a daily addiction to marijuana found CBD effective for his anxiety, enabling him to improve his sleep and quit marijuana usage. The patient's primary symptoms were erratic behavior, anxiety, poor sleep, and irritability. The patient was given 24 mg of CBD (administered as a spray) with six doses as needed during the day and two doses at bedtime. The dose was later lowered to 18 mg with six sprays during the day. The patient was evaluated monthly. He stopped marijuana use, experienced gradual reduction in anxiety and maintained a regular sleeping schedule. In addition, he was able to maintain a stable job and became more interactive with his family and friends[6] (Dr. Scott Shannon 2015).

Some may find it surprising that CBD from hemp is being using to treat marijuana addiction. Frequent marijuana use decreases the body's natural production and sensitivity to endocannabinoids. The withdrawal symptoms that someone with marijuana dependence experiences are caused by the artificially lowered endocannabinoids in their body from marijuana use. Withdrawal symptoms start within 24-48 hours and last up to three weeks, when the body restores its endocannabinoids. CBD is able to reduce THCs addictive effects and restore the endocannabinoids in the body.[7]

Chapter 9
Hemp CBD + Cocaine Addiction

"Remember that just because you hit bottom doesn't mean you have to stay there." Robert Downey Jr.

Cocaine is a powerful stimulant. It blocks dopamine transporters and stops the brain from removing excess dopamine. People trying to withdraw from cocaine experience fatigue, anxiety, irritability, agitation and paranoia.

Research on mice has found that CBD protects the mice from hepatotoxicity (chemical-driven liver damage) from cocaine[1] (Bornheim LM and Grillo MP 1998).

Since the endocannabinoid system is entangled with the neurobiology of cocaine addiction, Álvaro-Bartolomé and García-Sevilla evaluated the status of the CB1 and CB2 receptors, the endocytic cycle of CB1 receptors in the brain cortices of drug abusers and cocaine addicted rodents. They found that in cocaine addicted rats the CB1 receptor protein in the prefrontal cortex was reduced by 44%, which indicates that the receptor has been desensitized. They found that the CB2 receptors were not altered by cocaine use. The CB1 receptor protein was reduced by 41-80% in rats and mice with chronic cocaine use. They found that CB1 signalling was dampened and that the impairment of the CB1 receptor by cocaine may contribute to the alternation of neuroplasticity and neurotoxicity of the brains of cocaine addicts[2] (Álvaro-Bartolomé M and García-Sevilla JA 2013).

For cocaine use, CBD has mixed results. A study by Gerdeman et al found that neither CBD alone, nor a 1:1 ratio of THC:CBD reversed the sensitization effect of cocaine, which is the augmented motor-stimulant response what occurs with repeated use of a drug that is part of the drug craving and relapse cycle[3] (Gerdeman et al 2008).

A rat study by Luján et al found that acute administration of injected CBD had only a minimal effect on cocaine intake and relapse. In the study, they set out to determine if CBD could reduce cocaine reinforcement in mice. They found that CBD reduced voluntary cocaine consumption but did not reduce drug-induced reinstatement[4] (Luján et al 2018). CBD does not create euphoric or hedonic responses.

Between 2012 and 2015, Socias et al conducted a study observing 122 participants who reported that they were intentionally using cannabis to reduce their use of crack cocaine use. They found that cannabis use did successfully decrease the frequency of crack cocaine use in the participants[5] (Socias et al 2017).

In addition, there have been promising results, showing that CBD reduces the inflammation and seizures induced by cocaine[6] (Gobira et al 2015).

Chapter 10
Hemp CBD + Meth Addiction

"Numbing the pain for a while will make it worse
when you finally feel it." Albus Dumbledore

Methamphetamine, also known as meth and crystal meth, is an addictive stimulant. According to the 2017 National Drug Threat Survey, 29.8% of responding agencies reported that methamphetamine was the greatest drug threat in their areas.[1] Meth addiction comes with severe side effects, including aggression, hallucinations paranoia, psychological issues and death.

A study was done by Hay et al using 32 male rats to investigate whether CBD could reduce the motivation of self-administered methamphetamine and relapse. The study found that 80 mg/kg of CBD reduced the motivation to self-administer methamphetamine and reduced relapse seeking behaviour[2] (Hay et al 2018).

Relapse is a huge concern, even after long periods of abstinence. There is a strong connection between sleep impairment and relapse. In a study of rats deprived of REM sleep, researchers sought to determine whether CBD would prevent meth relapse. They found that CBD suppressed meth-induced reinstatement even under conditions of stress[3] (Karimi-Haghighi and Haghparast 2018).

The research is in the really early stages, while promising

there is a lot of work left to be done when it comes to the use of hemp CBD and meth addiction.

Chapter 11
Hemp CBD + Caffeine Addiction

"I have measured out my life with coffee spoons." T. S. Eliot

Caffeine is a central nervous system stimulant. Over 90% of American adults are regular consumers of caffeine. Americans consume an average of 200 mg of caffeine per day. For most people, caffeine is a habit that causes no harm, but it can become an addiction. Tolerance to caffeine can happen just as with drugs and alcohol—causing the user to need more and more caffeine to produce the same alertness.[1]

Withdrawal symptoms, cravings and relapse are common. Withdrawal symptoms generally start 12-24 hours after the cessation of caffeine and lasts between two and nine days. Typical withdrawal symptoms include changes in blood pressure, fatigue, irritability, difficulty concentrating, muscle or joint pain, constipation, abdominal pain and nausea[2] (Nicole Richter).

The American Psychiatric Association does not recognize caffeine addiction as a substance disorder; however, it does recognize caffeine *withdrawal* as a clinical condition. Yet, in 2012 the World Health Organization established caffeine addiction as a clinical disorder.[3]

Caffeine closely resembles the molecule adenosine and fits into the receptors for adenosine in the brain. Adenosine normally goes into the receptors and produces the feeling of fatigue but when caffeine molecules block the receptors, they prevent tiredness until the caffeine is metabolized. The adenosine cues the adrenal glands to secrete adrenaline. With repeated use, the brain grows more adenosine receptors in an attempt to maintain homeostasis.[4] Also, caffeine binding to the adenosine receptors causes blood vessels to dilate[5] (Nicole Richter).

Caffeine also causes a surge in dopamine in the brain—but not one that is as unbalanced as other drugs. The dopamine works more effectively when the adenosine receptors are blocked.[6]

In the midst of researching for this book I decided to run an unofficial study on myself. I have a long and sorted history with caffeine. I love coffee. I mean I *really* love it, but it doesn't love me. When I build up a tolerance and need more caffeine, I start getting brutal headaches that historically wake me up at 4 a.m. from caffeine withdrawals. This cycle forces me to quit caffeine and face, at the very least, a debilitatingly long weekend of headaches that sometimes last up to a week. While I suffer the withdrawals, I always swear that this is the last time I am getting on this caffeine addiction train—only to relapse in the midst of some other crazy work week cycle. After all, I am self-employed!

So while I was working on this book, I had built up my tolerance and had to quit again. I was so impressed with the results topical CBD showed in my withdrawal symptoms that I decided to systematically use both topical and internal hemp CBD to deal with quitting. I took 35 mg of Ology Essentials Full Spectrum Hemp CBD three times per day for seven days. I started the dosing on the day prior to ceasing caffeine. I also took a hot bath with 66 mg Ology Essential Bath Bombs for seven nights in a row. And I applied Vitality CBD Serum to my shoulders, neck and temples proactively two times per day for seven days.

The result was that I had a mild headache 24 hours after quitting caffeine that ceased when I applied Vitality CBD Serum to my neck and temples. That was it. One headache. I had set the entire weekend aside to suffer. It wasn't a double blind with a placebo group or anything like that—it was an information trial of one person. But as the one who avoided suffering, I am incredibly impressed with my results.

Chapter 12
Hemp CBD + Pain Management

"Although the world is full of suffering,
it is full also of the overcoming of it." Helen Keller

Let me just start out by saying that there is a time and a place for traditional medicine and prescription painkillers. I (Kayla) am not against the use of traditional pain management. I, personally, don't like the feeling of being on prescriptions for pain. I have lived in chronic pain since I was 16 years old. I thought it was from a car accident that never healed right, which seemed to spread into new pain as the years progressed. But while I was in my 50's, I was diagnosed with Ehler's Danlos Syndrome, a connective tissue disorder that results in joint instability, which predisposes patients to macro-trauma (joint dislocation or bone fracture) and micro-trauma (small tears in fibers and connective tissue of the muscles, as well as sprained ligaments, strained muscles and overstretched tendons). This answered the *why* of my lifetime of pain but didn't take away the endless pain.

At the time that I discovered hemp CBD, I was living on high doses of anti-inflammatory drugs, had prescription painkillers for the worst days, got regular steroid shots in my feet and hips and used a variety of natural and herbal medicine. Nothing really ever fully relieved my pain—it was always there on the edge. Enter hemp CBD—and my life was changed.

Today, I rarely take anti-inflammatory drugs, and pain that was constant is very subdued. I haven't had a single steroid shot since I started using hemp CBD. Today, I use a combination of topical and internal hemp CBD to manage my pain.

There are three types of pain: neuropathic pain, acute pain and centralized pain. Neuropathic pain is caused by damage or inflammation of nerves. Acute (perception or sensation of pain) is caused by injury or tissue damage. And centralized pain is chronic-like pain caused by damage or disease from conditions, such as Ehler's Danlos syndrome, fibromyalgia and migraines.

The main reason people seek prescription opioids and cannabis is pain relief. Wiese and Wilson-Poe reported, "Interestingly, when given access to cannabis, individuals currently using opioids for chronic pain decrease their use of opioids by 40–60% and report that they prefer cannabis to opioids. Patients in these studies reported fewer side effects with cannabis than with their opioid medications (including a paradoxical improvement in cognitive function) and a better quality of life with cannabis use, compared to opioids. Despite the vast array of cannabis products and administration routes used by patients in states with medical cannabis laws, cannabis has been consistently shown to reduce the opioid dose needed to achieve desirable pain relief"[1] (Wiese and Wilson-Poe 2018).

Ironically, opiate drugs used commonly to reduce pain actually cause an increase in muscle aches and pain.[2] Dr. Alfred Clavel Jr. explains this phenomenon: "In the United States we've been taught to think that when we feel pain, a pill will make us feel better. That's true after you have surgery or an injury that will heal in a few days or weeks. But what many people don't know is that if you use opioid pills for four or more weeks, it makes you more sensitive to pain and that makes the pain worse.

"Opioids do provide relief by blocking pain. But then, your body reacts by increasing the number of receptors to try to get the pain signal through again. So when the drug wears off, a person will experience more pain for about three days. If they continue to take opioids, the pills become less and less effective. The pain keeps increasing not because of an injury, but due to the opioids themselves.

"In addition, our bodies have natural opioids called endorphins. If your body becomes used to opioid pain medication, its ability to create and use natural endorphins will decrease. This makes you lose the ability to reduce pain on your own"[3] (Dr. Alfred Clavel Jr.).

Tolerance causes the body to require more opioids for the same pain relief, which leads to withdrawal symptoms, which requires more opioids to stop the withdrawal, and so the cycle goes.

Research is promising for using CBD for pain management. Topical CBD products can be applied right to trouble areas so that the CBD can work directly where it is needed most. Ingesting CBD products orally causes CBD and other compounds to enter the blood stream, which elicits full-body effects, taking up to two hours or more before those effects are experienced. With CBD topical products, the healing compound and other hemp-derived nutrients are almost immediately absorbed directly through your skin, allowing them to target the affected area for quicker and more focused effects. The analgesic, anti-inflammatory and neuroprotective effects of hemp CBD work together for some impressive and sometimes shocking pain relief.

A study by Hammell et al showed that topical use of CBD significantly reduced joint swelling, improved mobility and reduced pain for rats with arthritis[4] (D.C. Hammell et al 2016).

The authors of "Non-psychotropic plant cannabinoids: new therapeutic opportunities from an ancient herb" wrote, "More recently, CBD was shown to be effective in well-established experimental models of analgesia, as well as in acute and chronic models of inflammation in rodents. It is believed that the analgesic effect of CBD is mediated, at least in part, by TRPV1 and that its anti-arthritic action is due to a combination of immunosuppressive and anti-inflammatory effects"[5] (Angelo A. Izzo et al 2009).

The National Institute of Health has defined the term *cannabidiol*, but I've added plain English translations on some of the key points related to pain management within this definition for better understanding. "Cannabidiol is a phytocannabinoid [naturally occurring cannabinoid] from *Cannabis* species, which is devoid [not possessing] of psychoactive [affecting the mind] activity, with analgesic [acting to relieve pain], anti-inflammatory, antineoplastic [acting to prevent, inhibit or halt the development of a neoplasm/tumor] and chemopreventive [use of a drug to slow or prevent the development of cancer] activities...The analgesic [acting to relieve pain] effect of CBD is mediated through the binding of this agent to and activation of CB1"[6] (U.S. National Institute of Health).

A study by Corroon and Phillips found that 62% of CBD users reported that they chose to use CBD to treat a medical condition. The top three medical conditions they used CBD for were pain, anxiety and depression. Approximately 36% reported that CBD works for their medical condition very well without other treatments, while only 4.3% reported that it did not work very well for their condition.[7]

There are a few downsides to the hemp CBD industry. The most glaring and disheartening is the flood of companies wanting in the market at all costs with no regard for quality, honesty or purity of their products. Could it be that those who didn't find relief didn't get a high-quality product? Or that CBD simply didn't work for them? It is impossible to know, but fake products are unfortunately rampant in the hemp CBD industry, but there are also countless great companies who are truly passionate about hemp.

So how do you tell the difference? Look for companies that fully disclose their third party tested Certificate of Analysis (CoA) for consumers either on their websites, or even better, with a QR code on the product, which allows you to access the CoA of the lot you have purchased. If a company you buy from will not provide a CoA linked to the lot code of the product that you have purchased, it is time to dump that company and find another. Demand transparency—consumers can force more companies in the hemp industry to self-regulate.

There are also a lot of cheap products on the market. This can mean that it contains no CBD, it has a low dose of CBD, it is CBD from China or the dosage is inaccurately labeled. Just as jasmine and rose are expensive in the aromatherapy industry, so is hemp CBD. The prices are coming down, but not to the rock bottom prices that can be found at gas stations and on some websites. A good red flag to help you avoid companies in the market that are there just to make money is if the company makes miracle claims. That is a red flag that they don't know the basic rules of the FDA and the FTC. Claims change the intended use from a cosmetic to therapeutic, which makes it a drug. Brands cannot make claims to treat, prevent disease or affect the structure or function of the body without transforming their product into a drug. This is a basic fact that businesses in the industry have the responsibility to know—and if they don't know the basics, then what else don't they know about safety, purity, testing and quality?

The National Academics of Sciences Engineering Medicine concluded that, "there is conclusive or substantial evidence that cannabis or cannabinoids are effective: for the treatment for chronic pain in adults (cannabis), antiemetics in the treatment of chemotherapy-induced nausea and vomiting (oral cannabinoids), and for improving patient-reported multiple sclerosis spasticity symptoms (oral cannabinoids)."[8]

Chapter 13
Hemp CBD + Mental Health

"Every time you are tempted to react in the same old way,
ask if you want to be a prisoner of the past or a pioneer of the future."
Deepak Chopra

Many people turn to alcohol and drugs as a means to escape or self-medicate due to a very real mental health struggle. Wouldn't it be amazing to turn to non-addictive hemp CBD to self-medicate instead of an addictive substance? But words of caution: never, ever, ever stop your medication without consulting your doctor first.

Anxiety

"I promise you nothing is as chaotic as it seems.
Nothing is worth diminishing your health.
Nothing is worth poisoning yourself into stress, anxiety, and fear."
Steve Maraboli

Anxiety is your body's natural response to stress. However, anxiety disorder is an almost ever-present feeling of stress and fear that interferes with your life and can be debilitating. The common forms of anxiety disorders include panic disorder, phobia, social anxiety disorder, obsessive-compulsive disorder, separation anxiety disorder, illness anxiety disorder and post-traumatic stress disorder.

The Director of the National Institute on Drug Abuse, Nora D. Volkow, presented to the Senate Caucus on International Narcotics Control and stated that, "CBD has shown therapeutic efficacy in a range of animal models of anxiety and stress, reducing both behavioral and physiological (e.g., heart rate) measures of stress and anxiety. In addition, CBD has shown efficacy in small human laboratory and clinical trials. CBD reduced anxiety in patients with social anxiety subjected to a stressful public speaking task. In a laboratory protocol designed to model post-traumatic stress disorders, CBD improved 'consolidation of extinction learning,' in other words, forgetting of traumatic memories"[1] (Nora D. Volkow 2015).

I've (Kayla) spoken to countless people who've reported that they use hemp CBD for their anxiety. The self-reported results are nothing short of miraculous.

Depression

"At times, I feel overwhelmed and my depression leads me into darkness."
Dorothy Hamill

Depression, also known as Major Depressive Disorder, causes feelings of sadness and loss of interest in activities, which last for two weeks or more, but is very different from the experience of grief. Depression affects one in fifteen adults.

A report by de Mello Schier et al found that cannabidiol has antidepressant-like and anxiolytic-like (anxiety reducing) effects. In a 2011 study, twenty rats were treated with CBD in different doses of either imipramine (a tricyclic antidepressant) or a placebo of a saline solution. They found that a 30 mg/kg dosage of CBD had similar effects to the anti-depressant imipramine.[2]

The Depression Alliance has said that CBD has been found to be an effective treatment for depression and significantly improves depressive symptoms. The Depression Alliance explains, "CBD has been found to help improve depressive symptoms by modulating the actions of the endocannabinoids and also potentiating the effects of serotonin by enhancing the activity of the receptors unto which serotonin binds… Individuals with depression can begin with a dose of 5 to 10mg daily until the desired results are achieved."[3]

Post-Traumatic Stress Disorder (PTSD)

"Triggers are like little psychic explosions that crash through avoidance and bring the dissociated, avoided trauma suddenly, unexpectedly, back into consciousness."
Carolyn Spring

The American Psychiatric Association defines PTSD as, "A psychiatric disorder that can occur in people who have experienced or witnessed a traumatic event such as a natural disaster, a serious accident, a terrorist act, war/combat, rape, or other violent personal assault."[4]

Researcher from NYU Langone Medical Center found that people with PTSD have a low level of anandamide. As mentioned in Chapter 4, anandamide (AEA) is an endocannabinoid produced in the body. Health Care in America reported that, "These cannabinoids play a critical role in assisting PTSD cases by preventing the retrieval of the underlying trauma, effectively preventing traumatic memories and nightmares, while also helping attain emotional wellbeing"[5] (Angelique Moss 2018).

In a study be Elms et al, 91% of the PTSD patients who took CBD found experienced decreased PTSD symptoms.[6] The Veterans Association (VA) has said, "The VA published in 2016 that 66,000 veterans received treatment for opioid addiction. Cannabidiol (CBD) alleviates pain, diminishes inflammation, enhances mood, and is an effective remedy for a variety of other ailments, both physical and mental. CBD can probably be an alternative for opioids for military veterans with PTSD and related depressive symptoms. CBD has already shown positive results for these symptoms…There are several clinical trials and tons of anecdotal evidence on the effectiveness of CBD for helping with many of the difficulties our veterans are currently facing. From helping to relieve symptoms of PTSD, anxiety, chronic pain and more, CBD is becoming a popular choice for many veterans."[7]

Attention-Deficit/Hyperactivity Disorder (ADHD)

"Having ADD is like having a rocket ship brain but with bicycle brakes." Dr. Ed Hallowell

According to the American Psychiatric Association attention-deficit/hyperactivity disorder (ADHD) is one of the most common mental disorders affecting children that also persists into adulthood. The symptoms of ADHD include inattention, hyperactivity and impulsivity.[8] Treatment plans can include stimulants, non-stimulants, parent training, behavioral therapy and sometimes the use of off-label antidepressants. Patients suffering from ADHD have low dopamine levels in their prefrontal cortex of their brains. In good news, hemp CBD works to create a balanced level of neurotransmitter dopamine in the brain.

There is conflicting information about whether children on ADHD stimulant medications are at a higher risk for addiction. We will share both sides of the debate, but it is important to note that stimulant drugs like Ritalin, Adderall and Dexedrine are stimulants that increase the level of dopamine levels in the brain. As discussed in Chapter 3, dopamine plays an important role in addiction. Addictive substances release artificially high levels of dopamine in the brain, which can increase cravings by releasing artificially high levels of dopamine.

What is not up for debate is that patients with ADHD are 6.2 times more likely to develop a substance abuse disorder at younger ages, and up to 45% of adults with ADHD have abused or been addicted to alcohol abuse, while up to 30% have a history of illegal drug abuse or dependence. The question is *why*—is this increased risk for addiction caused by ADHA or by the use of stimulant drugs as young as six years old? Some studies have suggested that it is ADHD symptoms, such as impulsivity, poor inhibition, dopamine dysfunction and novelty-seeking behavior, that predispose a person to addiction. Also, those who have ADHD in addition to other mental health disorders, such as oppositional defiant disorder, bipolar disorder or conduct disorder, are estimated to be 8.8 times more likely to have a substance abuse disorder before age 18 compared with those with ADHD alone.[9]

A study by Lambert et al of 218 patients with ADHD and 182 without ADHD found that the duration of stimulant treatment impacted cocaine dependence. They found that 27% of ADHD patients who were exposed to stimulants for more than one year abused cocaine, compared to 15% of untreated patients.[10] Another study by Biederman et al of 109 children who were treated with stimulant medications between the ages of 7 and 12 years old had no significant difference in addictive behaviors as adults.[11] And still other studies are showing that those who are treated with stimulant medications are less likely to develop addictive behavior. The abuse of ADHD stimulant medications has been reported to be a problem for 9% of patients in grade school and high school, and for 35% of college aged patients.[12]

There have not been large scale research studies on the use of CBD for ADHD, however, there is an abundance of antidote reports and some case studies. A study by Cooper et al of 30 adults with ADHD using the cannabinoid medication, Sativex Oromucosal spray, showed an improvement in cognitive performance, hyperactivity, inattention and impulsive symptoms, with no detrimental effects.[14]

The antidote story, "We Give CBD Oil To Our Sons With ADHD," on Scary Mommy by Nicole Emanuel tells of their family's use of CBD for their child with oppositional defiance disorder and ADHD. Emanuel wrote, "After about a year on the medication [Adderall], a good friend of mine whose daughter also struggled to find balance with her ADHD and ODD, recommended we consider CBD oil. We had read several articles, including testimonies from adults with ADHD, as well as parents with children fighting the disorder, who had found great success using CBD." After working to find the right dosage for their 3 year old and 6 year old (who is taking Adderall) sons Emanuel reported, "We have seen such a positive change in both of our boys since we established a healthy routine of CBD oil in their daily regimen. Our oldest son, Brennden, has not been able to stop taking his Adderall just yet, because the medication helps him focus in ways I am not sure CBD oil will ever offer him. Nonetheless, we have been able to reduce his Adderall milligram use per day. CBD oil has been incredible for our family. Not only has it helped our children in many ways, but both my husband and I have been able to use CBD to reduce anxiety, stress, and pain relief." Nicole Emanuel says that CBD, combined with support and services from a therapist as well as a small dosage of Adderall, have her kids experiencing better sleep, balanced moods, improved appetites and eating habits, as well as less tantrums with faster de-escalation, more focus at school and healthier relationships.[15]

Consumer Reports shared that in October 2018 Lindsey Elliott gave her eleven-year-old son a 15 mg daily dose of CBD for his ADHD. Elliot reported that, "Tyler has improved leaps and bounds. Both he and his teacher have noticed a big difference. Tyler feels like he can concentrate more, and he feels more part of the team because he's not sitting there lost."[16]

Epilogue
by Carlton Bone

"You can't get clean, because you were never dirty"

Much has been said about how hemp can help a variety of addictive behaviors. As discussed in chapter three, and demonstrated through the stories of Keegan and Kayla, Substance Use Disorder is a shared chemical phenomenon with diverse effects. Each person's struggle is their own, and what strategies are going to be effective are going to vary. Fundamental to the success of all strategies is the de-stigmatization of those with Substance Use Disorder. Fear and stigma are at the root of chaotic drug use—a reality that, combined with the criminalization of certain drugs, creates and marginalizes those who find themselves in the grips of addiction.

Many individuals have found support for their sobriety through the integration of hemp-based CBD products. However, every road to recovery is predicated on the will and desire of an individual to address their drug use. Ultimately, the continued stigmatization of drug users and criminalization of drug use are the largest barrier to supporting drug user health. When drug use becomes a matter of survival, or perceived survival, then associated criminality is not a choice but a socially imposed consequence on certain drug users.

We don't hold the diabetic morally accountable for needing insulin, however, we are content to allow the individual with chronic pain who uses illicit opiates to be criminalized for what is fundamentally the same. Moreover, when the person with chronic pain ended up using opiates due to a lack of access to healthcare—an all too common problem in the U.S.—is it not a failure of the system to prevent their self-victimization? People are fundamentally biological beings, and beyond just getting well, we are pleasure driven beings. Our attitudes towards pleasure must therefore be as diverse as the substances that can make us feel good.

As outlined in Chapter 4, the body has an endocannabinoid system that is vital to its homeostatic operations. Substance Use Disorder chemically imbalances bodies, effects dependent on what substance is being abused and how, making the endocannabinoid system a critical site for understanding and addressing addictive behavior. While the information in the book is well suited for individual looking for guidance in how CBD can support their journey to sobriety, the endocannabinoid system may offer broader guidance on how we can reshape our attitude towards drug users, especially cannabinoid consumption.

Harm reduction is a set of practical strategies and ideas aimed at reducing negative consequences associated with drug use as well as a movement for social justice built on a belief in, and respect for, the rights of people who use drugs. Harm reduction incorporates a spectrum of strategies—from safer use, to managed use, to abstinence, to meeting drug users *where they're at*,—addressing conditions of use along with the use itself. In context of cannabinoids, the idea of harm reduction is multifaceted. For instance, Kayla and Keegan's use of CBD during their recovery underscores how cannabinoids can be a safer substitute to many other drugs. Indeed, this view is the extension of the breadth of evidence presented throughout this book as well as the belief of many leading experts in public health policy.[1]

The value of cannabinoids like CBD as tools in the harm reduction toolbox cannot be understated. As an alternative pain treatment, cannabinoids can save lives[2], while CBD has several therapeutic properties on its own that could indirectly be useful in the treatment of addiction disorders, such as its protective effect on stress vulnerability and neurotoxicity.[3] Moreover, the physiological role of the endocannabinoid system as a kind of internal harm reduction system reinforces the broader potential of cannabinoid therapies on a biological level. This view is espoused by Robert Melamede in a 2005 article published in the *Harm Reduction Journal*, who clarifies,

> "[A]ppropriate cannabis use reduces biological harm caused by biochemical imbalances, particularly those that increase in frequency with age. Proper cannabis use, as distinguished from misuse, may have significant positive health effects associated with the way cannabis mimics natural cannabinoids. In essence, it is proposed that the endocannabinoid system, selected by 600 million years of evolution, is a central mediator of biological harm reduction through its homeostatic activities."[4]

As a set of beliefs and practices, harm reduction can be reinforced through our endocannabinoid systems and cannabinoid consumption. The potential to reduce the harms of Substance Use Disorder through integrating or replacing treatments with CBD, that has been recognized by so many, is also an opportunity to critically engage with our assumptions about drug use across the board. The ability for individuals to make a shift in their drug use requires making our treatment more accessible, which can be done by meeting people where they are at. Listening to the lived experiences of those who have found guidance and support with CBD, like Kayla and Keegan, allows us to see the humanity that stereotypes of addiction can easily mask.

About The Authors

Kayla Fioravanti

Kayla Fioravanti is a certified aromatherapist, award-winning author, cosmetic formulator and hemp expert. In 1998 Kayla co-founded Essential Wholesale, which was listed as one of *INC Magazine's 5000 Fastest Growing Companies in America* three years in a row. Essential Wholesale began in Kayla's kitchen with a $50 investment in 1998 and sold for millions in 2011.

Kayla is a serial entrepreneur. After selling Essential Wholesale, she founded Selah Press, followed by the launch of Ology Essentials, which is a research-driven brand of high-quality hemp products, a fluffery-free aromatherapy certification program, an experience-based consulting business and an honest, no-hype custom formulating service. Ology Essentials is an indispensable aromatherapy and natural products resource and supplier. Kayla is an approved school educator by the National Association of Holistic Aromatherapists.

Kayla's writing is a sincere reflection of who she is. She writes everything from poetry to textbooks used in natural medicine programs. Kayla loves to research complex problems, dissect the information to its smallest component and then write it for her readers in everyday English.

Kayla's books include: *Hemp 101, A Little Handbook about Topical CBD: A Revolutionary Ingredient for the Skincare World, The*

Unspoken Truth About Essential Oils with Stacey Haluka, *The Art, Science and Business of Aromatherapy*, *DIY Kitchen Chemistry* and *How to Make Melt & Pour Soap Base from Scratch,* along with seven other books available on Amazon.

Kayla lives in Franklin, Tennessee with her family and a whole host of critters. She can be found at Ology Essentials working diligently on innovative formulations, supporting other small businesses as they enter the hemp CBD industry and building a family-based business with Keegan and Haleigh Fioravanti, along with the rest of the Ology Essentials team. You can find Kayla at OlogyEssentials.com and KaylaFioravanti.com.

Keegan Fioravanti

Keegan made Nashville his home in 2012. And while it was a far cry from his hometown of Portland, Oregon, he saw beauty in this southern city. Raised in a family of entrepreneurs, one could say Keegan was destined for this life. In fact, he co-owns Ology Essentials with his mom! Keegan started out as a hemp advocate for its uses in sustainable development, but when CBD came on the scene and changed his daily life, he knew he had to spread the good word.

Carlton Bone

Carlton Bone is the founder of the Upward Cannabis Kitchen, a state licensed manufacturer of cannabis infused edibles, as well as a partner of Dr. Melanie Bone, a licensed cannabis physician and educator. Beyond cannabis, Carlton is a passionate member of the harm reduction group, the Portland People's Outreach Project—a need based needle exchange working to improve the health and quality of life of houseless drug users—and a big opponent of the War on Drugs. When not writing and speaking about issues related to harm reduction, Carlton is busy developing new product formulations and researching how to improve the experiences of cannabis and drug users alike.

Resources: Where to Find Help

Substance Abuse and Mental Health Services Administration: https://www.samhsa.gov/find-help/national-helpline

This Naked Mind, Control Alcohol by Annie Grace
The Alcohol Experiment, 30-Day, Alcohol-Free Challenge to Interrupt Your Habits and Help You Take Control by Annie Grace

Partnership for Drug-free Kids and Center on Addiction: https://drugfree.org/landing-page/get-help-support/

The Surgeon General's Call to Action To Prevent and Reduce Underage Drinking. Appendix B: DSM-IV-TR Diagnostic Criteria for Alcohol Abuse and Dependence. https://www.ncbi.nlm.nih.gov/books/NBK44358/

National Institute on Alcohol Abuse and Alcoholism. Alcohol Facts and Statistics. https://www.niaaa.nih.gov/alcohol-facts-and-statistics

DSM-5 Criteria for Alcohol Use Disorder
https://www.niaaa.nih.gov/publications/brochures-and-fact-sheets/alcohol-use-disorder-comparison-between-dsm

- Substance Abuse and Mental Health Services
- Administration
- Alcoholics Anonymous
- Narcotics Anonymous
- Celebrate Recovery

References

Introduction

[1]World Health Organization Expert Committee on Drug Dependence 2017. December 2017. Web. https://www.who.int/features/qa/cannabidiol/en/

[2]Bergamaschi, Mateus Machado; Queiroz, Regina Helena Costa; Zuardi, Antonio Waldo; Crippa, Jose Alexandre. Safety and Side Effects of Cannabidiol, a Cannabis sativa Constituent. Current Drug Safety. 2011. WEB. http://www.eurekaselect.com/75752/article

[3]Bergamaschi, Mateus Machado; Queiroz, Regina Helena Costa; Zuardi, Antonio Waldo; Crippa, Jose Alexandre. Safety and Side Effects of Cannabidiol, a Cannabis sativa Constituent. Current Drug Safety. 2011. WEB. http://www.eurekaselect.com/75752/article

[4]Patent US6630507B1 US Grant, US Department of Health and Human Services (HHS). Google Patent. Cannabinoids as antioxidants and neuroprotectants. 1998. WEB. https://patents.google.com/patent/US6630507B1/en

[5]Iffland, Kerstin and Grotenhermen, Franjo. Cannabis and Cannabinoid Research, Volume 2, No. 1. An Update on Safety and Side Effects of Cannabidiol: A Review of Clinical Data and Relevant Animal Studies. 2017. WEB. https://www.liebertpub.com/doi/full/10.1089/can.2016.0034

[6]Iffland, Kerstin and Grotenhermen, Franjo. Cannabis and Cannabinoid Research, Volume 2, No. 1. An Update on Safety and Side Effects of Cannabidiol: A Review of Clinical Data and Relevant Animal Studies. 2017. WEB. https://www.liebertpub.com/doi/full/10.1089/can.2016.0034

Chapter 1: Our Personal Battles

[1]National Institute on Alcohol Abuse and Alcoholism. Underage Drinking: Why Do Adolescents Drink, What Are the Risks, and How Can Underage Drinking Be Prevented? January 2006. https://pubs.niaaa.nih.gov/publications/AA67/AA67.htm

[2]Milne, A A,. *The Many Adventures of Winnie-the-pooh.* New York: Dell, 1926. Print.

[3]Walt Disney Pictures. *Pooh's Grand Adventure: The Search for Christopher Robin.* Movie. 1997.

Chapter 2: The Difference Between Marijuana + Hemp

[1]Ministry of Hemp. Hemp vs Marijuana; What Makes Hemp Different from Marijuana. Miji Media LLC. 2018. WEB. https://ministryofhemp.com/hemp/not-marijuana/

[2]West, David Ph.D. North American Industrial Hemp Council. Hemp Myths and Realities. Ecomall. https://www.ecomall.com/greenshopping/hempmyths.htm

[3]Leaf Science. 5 Differences Between Hemp and Marijuana. 2014. WEB. https://www.leafscience.com/2014/09/16/5-differences-hemp-marijuana/

[4]Rothenberg, Erik. A Renewal of Common Sense, The Case for Hemp in 21st Century America. Vote Hemp, INC. 2001. WEB. https://www.votehemp.com/wp-content/uploads/2018/09/renewal.pdf

[5]Jacknin, Jeanette. Cannabinoids in Hemp for Beauty, Skin Health. Natural Products Insider. 2016. WEB. https://www.naturalproductsinsider.com/beauty/cannabinoids-hemp-beauty-skin-health

[6]MSMV News. News 4. Murfreesboro woman loses job after taking CBD. August 6, 2018. WEB. https://www.wsmv.com/news/murfreesboro-woman-loses-job-after-taking-cbd/video_b1bb68a3-5aab-5659-960b-575b53c17ba1.html

[7]Pappas, Robert PhD. 2018. Cannabis Confusion: Hemp, Marijuana, CBD and THC. Essential Oil University Facebook Page. WEB. https://www.facebook.com/note.php?note_id=10155147183928083

Chapter 3: Understanding Addiction

[1]CannabisMD. Addiction. https://cannabismd.com/health/addiction/

[2]Kemp, Cathryn. *Painkiller Addict: From wreckage to redemption - my true story.* Sphere. November 19, 2013.

[3]Prud'homme, Mélissa; Cata, Romulus; Jutras-Aswad1, Didier. "Cannabidiol as an Intervention for Addictive Behaviors: A Systematic Review of the Evidence." Web. May 21, 2015. https://www.ncbi.nlm.nih.gov/pmc/articles/PMC4444130/

[4]Grace, Annie. 2018. *This Naked Mind: Control Alcohol.* Avery, An Imprint of Penguin Random House. New York. Page 178.

[5]Noronha, Antonio B.C. et al. *Neurobiology of Alcohol Dependence.* Academic Press. 2014.

[6]Grace, Annie. 2018. *This Naked Mind: Control Alcohol.* Avery, An Imprint of Penguin Random House. New York. Pages 179-180.

[7]Grace, Annie. 2018. *This Naked Mind: Control Alcohol.* Avery, An Imprint of Penguin Random House. New York. Page 150.

[8]Grace, Annie. 2018. *This Naked Mind: Control Alcohol.* Avery, An Imprint of Penguin Random House. New York. Pages 178-180.

[9]Neuroscientifically Challenged. Know Your Brains: Nucleus Accumbens. Web. June 13, 2014. https://www.neuroscientificallychallenged.com/blog/2014/6/11/know-your-brain-nucleus-accumbens

Chapter 4: Cannabidiol + the Endocannabinoid System

[1]Grace, Annie. 2018. *This Naked Mind: Control Alcohol.* Avery, An Imprint of Penguin Random House. New York. Pages 43.

[2]Dustin Sulak, D.O. The Endocannabinoid System. Healer. 2016. WEB. https://healer.com/the-endocannabinoid-system/

[3]Rodolfo, Kevin. What is Homeostasis? Emeritus Professor Kelvin Rodolfo of the University of Illinois at Chicago's Department of Earth and Environmental Sciences provides this answer. WEB. https://www.scientificamerican.com/article/what-is-homeostasis/

[4]Russo, E.B. Clinical endocannabinoid deficiency (CECD): can this concept explain therapeutic benefits of cannabis in migraine, fibromyalgia, irritable bowel syndrome and other treatment-resistant conditions. PubMed. Us National Library of Medicine National Institute of Health. 2004. WEB. https://www.ncbi.nlm.nih.gov/pubmed/15159679

[5]The Recovery Village. "How Alcohol Affects the Cariovascular System. https://www.therecoveryvillage.com/alcohol-abuse/side-effects/alcohol-effects-cardiovascular-system/#gref

[6]National Institute on Drug Use. Advancing Addiction Science. "Health Consequences of Drug Misuse." March 2017. https://www.drugabuse.gov/publications/health-consequences-drug-misuse/cardiovascular-effects

[7]Editorial Staff. American Addiction Centers. "The Potential Repercussions of Substance Abuse on the Respiratory System." June 17, 2019. https://americanaddictioncenters.org/health-complications-addiction/respiratory-system

[8]Editorial Staff. American Addiction Centers. "The Potential Repercussions of Substance Abuse on the Respiratory System." June 17, 2019. https://americanaddictioncenters.org/health-complications-addiction/respiratory-system

[9]Davis, Jeanie Lerche. WebMD. "Drink Less for Strong Bones." https://www.webmd.com/osteoporosis/features/alcohol#1

[10]Editorial Staff. American Addiction Centers. "What Can Happen to the Renal

System as a Result of Excessive Drug Use?" October 17, 2019.
https://americanaddictioncenters.org/health-complications-addiction/renal-system

[11]Editorial Staff. American Addiction Centers. "How Can the Muscular System Be Harmed by the Effects of Drug Addiction?" September 3, 2019.
https://americanaddictioncenters.org/health-complications-addiction/muscular-system

[12]BreastCancer.org. Lower Your Risk Presents Breast Cancer Risk Factors. Drinking Alcohol. https://www.breastcancer.org/risk/factors/alcohol.

[13]ScienceNetLinks.com. Alcohol and the Human Body, The Endocrine System.
http://sciencenetlinks.com/interactives/alcohol/ebook/pages/endocrine-system.htm

[14]Editorial Staff. American Addiction Centers. "Why Is the Endocrine System at Risk from Substance Abuse?" June 17, 2019.
https://americanaddictioncenters.org/health-complications-addiction/endocrine-system

[15]Science Direct. Acetaldehyde.
https://www.sciencedirect.com/topics/pharmacology-toxicology-and-pharmaceutical-science/acetaldehyde

[16]Shavers, Brandon. Digestive Disease Specialists, Inc. "Alcohol Affects Digestive System, Unfolding Its True Side." January 15, 2019.
https://www.okddsi.net/blog/alcohol-affects-digestive-system-unfolding-its-true-side
[17]Editorial Staff. American Addiction Centers. "Health Concerns Related to the Digestive System from an Addiction to Drugs." June 17, 2019.
https://americanaddictioncenters.org/health-complications-addiction/digestive-system

[18]Alcohol Addiction Center. Effects of Alcohol.
https://alcoholaddictioncenter.org/alcohol/effects/

[19]Watkins, Meredith M.A., M.F.T. American Addiction Centers. "How Drugs Affect the Brain and Central Nervous System." September 11, 2019.
https://americanaddictioncenters.org/health-complications-addiction/central-nervous-system

[20]Editorial Staff. American Addiction Centers. "Why Is the Lymphatic System at Risk from Drug or Alcohol Abuse?" September 3, 2019.
https://americanaddictioncenters.org/health-complications-addiction/lymphatic-system

[21]Hurly, Adam. GQ Magazine. "Here's Exactly How Bad Drinking Alcohol Is for Your Skin." December 12, 2017. https://www.gq.com/story/how-bad-is-drinking-alcohol-for-your-skin

[22]Editorial Staff. American Addiction Centers. "What Drug Abuse Can Do to the Skin." June 17, 2019. https://americanaddictioncenters.org/health-complications-addiction/drugs-skin

[23]Science Daily. "Alcoholics' Deficits In Smell Are Linked To Frontal Lobe Dysfunction." July 25, 2006. https://www.sciencedaily.com/releases/2006/07/060725092208.htm

[24]Clason, Debbie. Healthy Hearing. "Drinking and Hearing loss." July 6, 2017. https://www.healthyhearing.com/report/52762-Drinking-and-hearing-loss

[25]Dotinga, Randy. Health Day. News for Healthier Living. "Painkillers May have Caused Limbaugh's Deafness." October 16, 2003. https://consumer.healthday.com/general-health-information-16/drug-abuse-news-210/painkillers-may-have-caused-limbaugh-s-deafness-515577.html

[26]Pubs.niaa.nih.gov. Medical Consequences. "Alcohol and the Immune System. "https://pubs.niaaa.nih.gov/publications/10report/chap04b.pdf

[27]Staff Writer. Serenity at Summit. "How Drugs and Alcohol Affect the Immune System." https://www.serenityatsummit.com/alcohol-addiction/drugs-alcohol-affect-immune-system/

[28]Hewitt, Robin. Livestrong. "How Does Alcohol Affect the Reproductive System?" https://www.livestrong.com/article/19016-alcohol-affect-reproductive-system/

[29]Hurt, Lukas. Leafly. "Meet Lumir Hanus, Who Discovered the First Endocannabinoid." December 13, 2016. https://www.leafly.com/news/science-tech/lumir-hanus-discovered-first-endocannabinoid-anandamide

[30]Healthline. "A Simple Guide to the Endocannabinoid System." https://www.healthline.com/health/endocannabinoid-system-2

[31]Gómez, Paul. Prof of Pot. "Does CBD Block the High of THC." June 23, 2017. https://profofpot.com/does-cbd-block-high-of-thc/

[32]Chye, Yann et al. US National Library of Medicine, National Institutes of Health. "The Endocannabinoid System and Cannabidiol's Promise for the Treatment of Substance Use Disorder." February 19, 2019.

[33]Bone, Dr. Melanie. Personal Communication. November 3, 2019.

Chapter 5: Hemp CBD + Alcohol Addiction

[1]Her View from Her Home. Facebook post. May 27, 2019. https://www.facebook.com/kayla.fioravanti/posts/10217025369098955

[2]Foundation for a Drug-Free World, Find out the Truth about Drugs. "The Truth About Alcohol." https://www.drugfreeworld.org/real-life-stories/alcohol.html.

[3]BreastCancer.org. Lower Your Risk Presents Breast Cancer Risk Factors. Drinking Alcohol. https://www.breastcancer.org/risk/factors/alcohol.

[4]Grace, Annie. 2018. *This Naked Mind: Control Alcohol.* Avery, An Imprint of Penguin Random House. New York. Page 190.

[5]Grace, Annie. 2018. *This Naked Mind: Control Alcohol.* Avery, An Imprint of Penguin Random House. New York. Page 37.

[6]JAMA Psychiatry. "Prevalence of 12-Month Alcohol Use, High-Risk Drinking, and DSM-IV Alcohol Use Disorder in the United States, 2001-2002 to 2012-2013: Results From the National Epidemiologic Survey on Alcohol and Related Conditions." September 2017. Web. https://jamanetwork.com/journals/jamapsychiatry/fullarticle/2647079

[7]Nutt, David J. Prof.; King, Leslie A.; Phillips, Lawrence D. PhD. The Lancet. Drug harms in the UK: a multicriteria decision analyses. November 01, 2010. https://www.thelancet.com/journals/lancet/article/PIIS0140-6736(10)61462-6/fulltext

[8]National Institute on Alcohol Abuse and Alcoholism. "Alcohol Facts and Statistics." Web. https://www.niaaa.nih.gov/alcohol-facts-and-statistics

[9]CDC. National Vital Statistics Reports. Deaths: Final Data 2013. February 16, 2016. Web. https://www.cdc.gov/nchs/data/nvsr/nvsr64/nvsr64_02.pdf

[10]American Addiction Centers Research. "Statistics & Information on Alcoholism & Addiction Treatment Help." July 3, 2019. Web. https://www.alcohol.org/statistics-information/

[11]Gonzalez-Cuevas et al. Nature. "Unique treatment potential of cannabidiol for the prevention of relapse to drug use: preclinical proof of principle." March 22, 2018. https://www.nature.com/articles/s41386-018-0050-8

[12]Liput, Daniel J. et al. Science Direct. Pharmacology Biochemistry and Behavior. "Transdermal delivery of cannabidiol attenuates binge alcohol-induced neurodegeneration in a rodent model of an alcohol use disorder." October 2013. Web. https://www.sciencedirect.com/science/article/pii/S0091305713002104

[13]Grace, Annie. 2018. *This Naked Mind: Control Alcohol.* Avery, An Imprint of Penguin Random House. New York. Page 37.

[14]Zou, Shenglong and Kumar, Ujendra. US National Library of Medicine, National Institutes of Health. "Cannabinoid Receptors and the Endocannabinoid System: Signaling and Function in the Central Nervous System." March 19, 2018. Web. https://www.ncbi.nlm.nih.gov/pmc/articles/PMC5877694/

Chapter 6: Hemp CBD + Nicotine Addiction

[1]Addiction Center. "Nicotine Addiction and Abuse. A nicotine addiction is one of the hardest addictions to break, yet over 1 million tobacco users quit every year." Web. https://www.addictioncenter.com/nicotine/

[2]Allar, Daniel. Cardiovascular Business. Alternate addiction: 1.9 million US e-cig users have never smoked cigarettes. October 10, 2018 Web. https://www.cardiovascularbusiness.com/topics/healthcare-economics/19m-us-e-cig-users-have-never-smoked-cigarettes

[3]Morgan ,CJ et al. . US National Library of Medicine, National Institutes of Health. "Cannabidiol reduces cigarette consumption in tobacco smokers: preliminary findings." September 2013. Web. https://www.ncbi.nlm.nih.gov/pubmed/23685330

[4]Hindocha C et al. US National Library of Medicine, National Institutes of Health. "Cannabidiol reverses attentional bias to cigarette cues in a human experimental model of tobacco withdrawal." May 1, 2018. Web. https://www.ncbi.nlm.nih.gov/pubmed/29714034

[5]Chye et al. US National Library of Medicine, National Institutes of Health. "The Endocannabinoid System and Cannabidiol's Promise for the Treatment of Substance Use Disorder." February 2019. Web. https://www.ncbi.nlm.nih.gov/pmc/articles/PMC6390812/

Chapter 7: Hemp CBD + Opioid Addiction

[1]National Institute on Drug Abuse. Opioid Overdose Crisis. Revised January 2019. Web. https://www.drugabuse.gov/drugs-abuse/opioids/opioid-overdose-crisis

[2]Wiese, Beth and Wilson-Poe, Adrianne R. "Emerging Evidence for Cannabis' Role in Opioid Use Disorder." Cannabis and Cannabinoid Research. Volume 3.1, 2018.

[3]Katsidoni, Anagnostou, and Panagis. US National Library of Medicine, National Institutes of Health. " Cannabidiol inhibits the reward-facilitating effect of morphine: involvement of 5-HT1A receptors in the dorsal raphe nucleus." March 2013. https://www.ncbi.nlm.nih.gov/pubmed/22862835

[5]Peachman, Rachel Rabkin. Consumer Reports. "Can CBD Treat Opioid Addiction? The popular cannabis compound may help some people wean off addictive pain meds." April 23, 2019. Web. https://www.consumerreports.org/cbd/can-cbd-treat-opioid-addiction/

[6]Ren et al. US National Library of Medicine, National Institutes of Health. "Cannabidiol, a nonpsychotropic component of cannabis, inhibits cue-induced heroin seeking and normalizes discrete mesolimbic neuronal disturbances." November 2009. Web. https://www.ncbi.nlm.nih.gov/pubmed/19940171

[7]Bradford, Ashley C.; Bradford, David W. PhD; Abraham, Amanda, PhD et al. JAMA Network. JAMA Internal Medicine. "Association Between US State Medical Cannabis Laws and Opioid Prescribing in the Medicare Part D Population." Original Investigation Health Care Policy and Law. May 2018. Web.

References

https://jamanetwork.com/journals/jamainternalmedicine/fullarticle/2676999

[8]Wiese, Beth and Wilson-Poe, Adrianne R. "Emerging Evidence for Cannabis' Role in Opioid Use Disorder." Cannabis and Cannabinoid Research. Volume 3.1, 2018.

[9]Bone, Carlton. "Building Out Our Toolbox: Notes on Integrative Care with Cannabinoids and Opioids", CBD Health & Wellness Magazine, January/February 2019 Issue.

Chapter 8: Hemp CBD + Marijuana Addiction
[1]Hasin DS, Saha TD, Kerridge BT, et al. Prevalence of Marijuana Use Disorders in the United States Between 2001-2002 and 2012-2013. *JAMA Psychiatry.* 2015;72(12):1235-1242. doi:10.1001/jamapsychiatry.2015.1858

[2]UK Research and Innovation. "Cannabidiol: a novel treatment for cannabis dependence?" Lead Research Organisation: University College London. Department Name: Clinical Health and Educational Psych. Web. https://gtr.ukri.org/project/0264FAF2-1CE1-4894-BE33-C53A27E49217

[3]National Institute on Drug Abuse. Advancing Addiction Science. "Is Marijuana Addictive?" Web. https://www.drugabuse.gov/publications/research-reports/marijuana/marijuana-addictive

[4]Crippa et al. US National Library of Medicine, National Institutes of Health. "Cannabidiol for the treatment of cannabis withdrawal syndrome: a case report." April 2013. Web. https://www.ncbi.nlm.nih.gov/pubmed/23095052

[5]Babalonis et al. US National Library of Medicine, National Institutes of Health. "Oral cannabidiol does not produce a signal for abuse liability in frequent marijuana smokers." March 2017. Web. https://www.ncbi.nlm.nih.gov/pubmed/28088032

[6]Shannon, Scott MD and Opila-Lehman, Janet MD. US National Library of Medicine, National Institutes of Health. "Cannabidiol Oil for Decreasing Addictive Use of Marijuana: A Case Report." December 2015. Web. https://www.ncbi.nlm.nih.gov/pmc/articles/PMC4718203/
[7]Richter, Nicole. Marijuana Break. "CBD for Drug Addiction: How One Can Use It [And How It Works]" Web. https://www.marijuanabreak.com/cbd-to-treat-drug-addiction-how-it-works-and-how-you-can-use-it

Chapter 9: Hemp CBD + Cocaine Addiction
[1]Bornheim LM and Grillo MP. US National Library of Medicine, National Institutes of Health. "Characterization of cytochrome P450 3A inactivation by cannabidiol: possible involvement of cannabidiol-hydroxyquinone as a P450 inactivator." October 1998. https://www.ncbi.nlm.nih.gov/pubmed/9778318

[2]Álvaro-Bartolomé M and García-Sevilla JA. US National Library of Medicine, National Institutes of Health. "Dysregulation of cannabinoid CB1 receptor and associated signaling networks in brains of cocaine addicts and cocaine-treated rodents." September 2013. Web. https://www.ncbi.nlm.nih.gov/pubmed/23727505

[3]Gerdeman GL, Schechter JB, French ED. US National Library of Medicine, National Institutes of Health. "Context-specific reversal of cocaine sensitization by the CB1 cannabinoid receptor antagonist rimonabant." October 2008. Web. https://www.ncbi.nlm.nih.gov/pubmed/18059436

[4]Luján MÁ, Castro-Zavala A, Alegre-Zurano L, Valverde O. US National Library of Medicine, National Institutes of Health. "Repeated Cannabidiol treatment reduces cocaine intake and modulates neural proliferation and CB1R expression in the mouse hippocampus." December 2018. Web. https://www.ncbi.nlm.nih.gov/pubmed/30273593

[5]Socias et al. US National Library of Medicine, National Institutes of Health. "Intentional cannabis use to reduce crack cocaine use in a Canadian setting: A longitudinal analysis." September 2017. https://www.ncbi.nlm.nih.gov/pubmed/28399488

[6]Gobira P.H., Vilela L.R., Gonçalves B.D., Santos R.P., de Oliveira A.C., Vieira L.B., Aguiar D.C., Crippa J.A., Moreira F.A. Cannabidiol, a Cannabis sativa constituent, inhibits cocaine-induced seizures in mice: Possible role of the mTOR pathway and reduction in glutamate release. Neurotoxicology. 2015;50:116–121. doi: 10.1016/j.neuro.2015.08.007.

Chapter 10: Hemp CBD + Meth Addiction

[1]U.S. Department of Justice Druge Enforcement Administration. "2017 National Drug Threat Assessment." October 2017. DEA-DCT-DIR-040-17. https://www.dea.gov/sites/default/files/2018-07/DIR-040-17_2017-NDTA.pdf

[2]Hay et al. Sage Journals. Journal of Psychopharmacology. Cannabidiol treatment reduces the motivation to self-administer methamphetamine and methamphetamine-primed relapse in rats. September 2018. Web. https://journals.sagepub.com/doi/abs/10.1177/0269881118799954

[3]Karimi-Haghighi S., Haghparast A. US National Library of Medicine, National Institutes of Health. "Cannabidiol inhibits priming-induced reinstatement of methamphetamine in REM sleep deprived rats." March 2018. Web. https://www.ncbi.nlm.nih.gov/pubmed/28870635

Chapter 11: Hemp CBD + Caffeine

[1]Addiction Center. Caffeine Addiction and Abuse. "What is Caffeine Addiction." Web. https://www.addictioncenter.com/stimulants/caffeine/

[2]Richter, Nicole. Marijuana Break. "Have a Caffeine Headache? Here's How Cannabis Might Be Able to Help." Web. https://www.marijuanabreak.com/can-cannabis-help-treat-caffeine-headaches

[3]Addiction Center. Caffeine Addiction and Abuse. "What is Caffeine Addiction." Web. https://www.addictioncenter.com/stimulants/caffeine/

[4]Addiction Center. Caffeine Addiction and Abuse. "What is Caffeine Addiction."

Web. https://www.addictioncenter.com/stimulants/caffeine/

[5]Richter, Nicole. Marijuana Break. "Have a Caffeine Headache? Here's How Cannabis Might Be Able to Help." Web. https://www.marijuanabreak.com/can-cannabis-help-treat-caffeine-headaches

[6]Addiction Center. Caffeine Addiction and Abuse. "What is Caffeine Addiction." Web. https://www.addictioncenter.com/stimulants/caffeine/

Chapter 12: Hemp CBD + Pain Management

[1]Wiese, Beth and Wilson-Poe, Adrianne R. "Emerging Evidence for Cannabis' Role in Opioid Use Disorder." Cannabis and Cannabinoid Research. Volume 3.1, 2018.

[2]Editorial Staff. American Addiction Centers. "How Can the Muscular System Be Harmed by the Effects of Drug Addiction?" September 3, 2019. https://americanaddictioncenters.org/health-complications-addiction/muscular-system

[3]Clavel, Alfred Dr. Jr. Health Partners. "Why Opioids make Pain Worse." https://www.healthpartners.com/blog/why-opioids-make-pain-worse/
[4]D.C. Hammell; L.P. Zhang; F. Ma; S.M. Abshire; S.L. McIlwrath; A.L. Stinchcomb; and K.N. Westlund. Transdermal cannabidiol reduces inflammation and pain-related behaviours in a rat model of arthritis. U.S. National Library of Medicine. National Institutes of Health. 2016. WEB. https://www.ncbi.nlm.nih.gov/pmc/articles/PMC4851925/

[5]Angelo A. Izzo; Francesca Borrelli; Raffaele Capasso; Vincenzo Di Marzo; and Raphael Mechoulam. Non-psychotropic plant cannabinoids: new therapeutic opportunities from an ancient herb. Cell Press. 2009. WEB. http://www.stcm.ch/en/files/paper_izzo_tips_2009.pdf

[6]National Institute of Health. U.S. National Library of Medicine. National Center for Biotechnology Information. PubChem. Open Chemistry Data Base. Compound Summary for CID 644019, Cannabidiol. WEB. https://pubchem.ncbi.nlm.nih.gov/compound/cannabidiol#section=Top

[7]Corroon, Jamie and Phillips, Joy A. US National Library of Medicine, National Institutes of Health. " A Cross-Sectional Study of Cannabidiol Users. July 1, 2018. https://www.ncbi.nlm.nih.gov/pmc/articles/PMC6043845/

[8]The National Academics of Sciences Engineering Medicine. Health and Medicine Division. "The Health Effects of Cannabis and Cannabinoids: The Current State of Evidence and Recommendations for Research." Committee's Conclusions. January 12, 2017.
http://nationalacademies.org/hmd/~/media/Files/Report%20Files/2017/Cannabis-Health-Effects/Cannabis-conclusions.pdf

Chapter 13: Hemp CBD for Anxiety, Depression + PTSD

[1]Volkow, Nora D. National Institute on Drug Abuse. Advancing Addiction Science.

"The Biology and Potential Therapeutic Effects of Cannabidiol." June 24, 2015. https://www.drugabuse.gov/about-nida/legislative-activities/testimony-to-congress/2015/biology-potential-therapeutic-effects-cannabidiol

[2]de Mello Schier, Alexandre R et al. CNS & Neuroligical Disorders. Drug Targets. "Antidepressant-Like and Anxiolytic-Like Effects of Cannabidiol: A Chemical Compound of Cannabis sativa." 2014. https://cbd-b.be/wp-content/uploads/2018/09/2014-Antidepressant-Like-and-Anxiolytic-Like-Effects-of-Cannabidiol.pdf

[3]Depression Alliance Staff. "CBD Oil: A Cure for Depression?" Depression Alliance. https://www.depressionalliance.org/cbd-oil/

[4]American Psychiatric Association. "What is Posttraumatic Stress Disorder?" https://www.psychiatry.org/patients-families/ptsd/what-is-ptsd

[5]Moss, Angelique. Healthcare in America. "Cannabis could be the key to treating people with PTSD." October 31, 2018. https://healthcareinamerica.us/cannabis-key-treating-ptsd-b4abf432215

[6]Elms, Lucas et al. Journal of Alternative and Complementary Medicine. "Cannabidiol in the Treatment of Post-Traumatic Stress Disorder: A Case Series ." April 1, 2019. https://www.ncbi.nlm.nih.gov/pmc/articles/PMC6482919/

[7]Veterans Association. "Can CBD Oil Help with Anxiety & PTSD In Veterans?" https://va.org/can-cbd-oil-help-with-anxiety-ptsd-in-veterans

[8]American Psychiatric Association. "What is ADHD?" https://www.psychiatry.org/patients-families/adhd/what-is-adhd

[9]Jain, Shailesh MD, MPH, ABDA. MD Edge Psychiatry. "Do stimulants for ADHD increase the risk of substance use disorders?" August 10, 2011. https://www.mdedge.com/psychiatry/article/64399/addiction-medicine/do-stimulants-adhd-increase-risk-substance-use-disorders#bib6

[10]Lambert NM, Hartsough CS. "Prospective study of tobacco smoking and substance dependencies among samples of ADHD and non-ADHD participants." J Learn Disabil. 1998;31(6):533-544.

[11]Biederman J, Monuteaux MC, Spencer T, et al. Stimulant therapy and risk for subsequent substance use disorders in male adults with ADHD: a naturalistic controlled 10-year follow-up study. Am J Psychiatry. 2008;165(5):597-603.

[12]Jain, Shailesh MD, MPH, ABDA. MD Edge Psychiatry. "Do stimulants for ADHD increase the risk of substance use disorders?" August 10, 2011. https://www.mdedge.com/psychiatry/article/64399/addiction-medicine/do-stimulants-adhd-increase-risk-substance-use-disorders#bib6

[13]Strohbeck-Kuehner, Peter et al. "Case report Cannabis improves symptoms of

ADHD." Cannabinoids 2008. http://cannabis-med.org/data/pdf/en_2008_01_1.pdf

[14]Cooper, Ruth E. et al. "Cannabinoids in attention-deficit/hyperactivity disorder: A randomized controlled trial." European Neuropsychopharmacology Volume 27, Issue 8, August 2017, Pages 795-808.
https://www.sciencedirect.com/science/article/abs/pii/S0924977X17302377

[15]Emanuel, Nicole. "We Give CBD Oil To Our Sons With ADHD." Scary Mommy.
https://www.scarymommy.com/shadow-discipline-dangerous/

[16]Peachman, Rachel Rabkin. "Can CBD Help Your Child? Parents are using the cannabis compound to manage hard-to-treat ailments in kids, but there are still many unknowns." Consumer Reports. February 26, 2019.
https://www.consumerreports.org/cbd/can-cbd-help-your-child

Epilogue
[1]Lucas, P. Rationale for cannabis-based interventions in the opioid overdose crisis. Harm Reduct J 14, 58 (2017) doi:10.1186/s12954-017-0183-9

[2]Collen M. Prescribing cannabis for harm reduction. Harm Reduct J. 2012; 9:1. Published 2012 Jan 1. doi:10.1186/1477-7517-9-1

[3]Prud'homme M, Cata R, Jutras-Aswad D. Cannabidiol as an Intervention for Addictive Behaviors: A Systematic Review of the Evidence. Subst Abuse. 2015; 9:33–38. Published 2015 May 21. doi:10.4137/SART.S25081

[4]Melamede, R. Harm reduction-the cannabis paradox. Harm Reduct J 2, 17 (2005) doi:10.1186/1477-7517-2-17